Elizabeth Hagan
Joan Gormley

HIV/AIDS and the Drug Culture
Shattered Lives

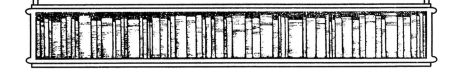

The Haworth Press, Inc.

HIV/AIDS
and the Drug Culture
Shattered Lives

HAWORTH Psychosocial Issues of HIV/AIDS
R. Dennis Shelby, PhD
Senior Editor

HIV and Social Work: A Practitioner's Guide edited by David M. Aronstein and Bruce J. Thompson

HIV/AIDS and the Drug Culture: Shattered Lives by Elizabeth Hagan and Joan Gormley

HIV/AIDS
and the Drug Culture
Shattered Lives

Elizabeth Hagan
Joan Gormley

The Haworth Press
New York • London

The Haworth Press, Inc., 10 Alice Street, Binghamton, NY 13904-1580

Cover design by Monica L. Seifert.

Library of Congress Cataloging-in-Publication Data

Hagan, Elizabeth, 1952-
    HIV/AIDS and the drug culture : shattered lives / Elizabeth Hagan, Joan Gormley.
        p.   cm.
    Includes bibliographical references (p.   ) and index.
    ISBN 0-7890-0465-8 (alk. paper).
    1. AIDS (Disease)—United States. 2. Drug abuse—United States. 3. Needle exchange pro-
grams. I. Gormley, Joan. II. Title.
RA644.25.H33   1998
362.1'969792'00973—dc21   98-6097
                                                                                                    CIP

CONTENTS

980942

ABOUT THE AUTHORS

Elizabeth Hagan, RN, BSN, ACRN, is Patient Care Coordinator at Hospice Care of Rhode Island in Pawtucket, Rhode Island. A registered nurse for twenty-five years, she initially became involved with AIDS patients through teaching home infusion therapies to patients and families in the early 1990s. In 1994, she joined Hospice Care of Rhode Island as a field nurse for the George Street Program, a team specializing in the care of patients with AIDS, and in 1996, she became Coordinator of the program. She has been a member of the Association of Nurses in AIDS Care since 1995 and became Board Certified as an AIDS Certified Registered Nurse (ACRN) in 1957.

Joan Gormley, RN, BSN, is Study Coordinator at the Immunology Center, The Miriam Hospital, in Providence, Rhode Island. She directs the care of patients with HIV in clinical trials. In 1992, she became a nurse clinician involved with approximately 400 HIV/AIDS patients. Her interest in working with injecting drug using patients has led her to participate in a pilot project on needle exchange, which was supported by the State of Rhode Island. Currently, she volunteers weekly on the local level in the needle exchange program and in a free clinic that addresses the medical and psychosocial needs of high-risk patients. She continues to fight at the national level for rescinding the federal ban on funds for needle exchange programs.

Preface

Most biographies and testimonials are written by a well-educated bereaved family member in honor of a loved one. From a review of the literature on the subject HIV/AIDS, the point of view and specialized needs of the dually diagnosed IV drug users with HIV/AIDS are underrepresented. As these people become immersed in the drug culture, common goals of careers and family are superseded by the need to meet the demands of the addiction. That is why intravenous drug use and addiction often result in the users becoming isolated from family and friends who might otherwise represent them by telling their stories; drug users are a population unable to write for themselves. Heroin changes the user's lifestyle and character, dismantling childhood value systems and opening doors to an unwelcome world with a culture all its own.

A diagnosis of HIV/AIDS can devastate the most ordered lives. Disclosing this diagnosis to a fragile individual struggling to cope with the myriad of issues associated with addiction is, indeed, life shattering. How can the angry, lonely individual who depends on the solace of heroin to meet the demands of a daily routine even begin to learn to accept a crippling disease?

This book evolved from years of repeated dealings with a large, metropolitan population of dually diagnosed intravenous drug users with HIV/AIDS. Smaller communities may lack this opportunity to treat and observe such a large, specialized group. As our programs have developed through specialization, we have benefited and received positive reinforcement. By focusing on the special needs of people with addictions, we have developed effective strategies to manage their complex care. It is only through exposure to and interaction with this population and its unique culture that the caregiver or clinician is able to identify certain patterns of behavior. From this viewpoint it is possible to begin to understand the underlying causes. As difficult and uncomfortable as this experience may be, the result is mutually beneficial: Patients benefit from anticipation of their needs; caregivers and clinicians benefit through personal and professional growth.

Another advantage found within a metropolitan area is the opportunity to tap into multiple community services. Part of the primary care provider's role is to initiate referrals. Medical services are only a portion of the complex needs of this population. Coordination of community services is necessary to encompass the scope of issues. Attempting to treat a dually diagnosed individual independently, in isolation, will short-change the patient and frustrate the provider.

The cooperation of all community agencies is essential for meeting the complex needs of this population. Cooperation will result in increased effectiveness and decreased duplication of services. The close communication and interaction we enjoy between the hospital-based clinic and the hospice home care agency has enabled patients to appreciate the importance of keeping in touch with the medical system. Through the sharing of concerns and successes, we have developed guidelines that meet the needs of the patient, the team, and the community.

The intention of this book is to provide information and guidance to clinicians and caregivers dealing directly with the challenge of the dually diagnosed HIV/AIDS and intravenous drug user, to assist in the development of comprehensive care and treatment plans, and to share what we have learned. We hope this information will help to prepare health care teams to deal with the frustrations inherent in this field. Although many medical centers, clinics, and home care agencies face identical concerns, they may deal with small numbers and lack the opportunity to develop effective strategies for dealing with these common issues. However, as AIDS becomes a chronic disease and the average life expectancy extends well into a second decade, the numbers of patients presenting with these problems increases. The situations and solutions presented in this book can be applied to any patient care setting.

Each case study explores an actual situation and individual, focusing on a particular problem. Both names and circumstances have been altered to ensure confidentiality. Each case study is followed by a correlating set of strategies that have proven safe and effective for managing the diverse and complex needs of this population. Part I is written from the point of view of the health care professionals in the outpatient clinic setting and addresses nursing, social work, and case management issues for care planning. Part II focuses on the same issues from the point of view of the home health care team. Part III identifies some of the challenges for the hospice care provider as the patients' needs change from palliative care to intensive symptom management and family/caregiver education and support. The principles of the harm reduction model are applicable across the continuum of care, enabling practitioners to provide options for change to individuals who might otherwise be lost within the health care system.

PART I:
MANAGEMENT FROM
THE OUTPATIENT CLINIC

Introduction

The Scope of the Issue

Facts about needle exchange programs, injection drug use,
and seroprevalence among intravenous drug users

At one time the interaction between injecting drug users and the health care system was limited to acute medical issues, such as cellulitis, pneumonia, endocarditis, and drug overdose. Health care providers gave little thought to an individual's chronic medical problems. The HIV epidemic dramatically changed this situation (Wartenberg and Samet, 1992).

One of the largest causes of HIV transmission in the United States is the sharing of needles and syringes for the injection of drugs. It has led to over 205,000 documented cases of AIDS. At least twice as many whites as African Americans inject drugs, but injection-related HIV transmission disproportionately affects communities of color. African-American and Latino communities face a public health crisis. If we combine data on AIDS and drug use, we find that among those who inject drugs, African Americans are four times as likely as whites to get AIDS (Day, 1997). In 1996 almost 100,000 African Americans had injection-related AIDS or had died from AIDS. AIDS is the leading cause of death among twenty-four to forty-four-year-old Latinos in the United States; more than half of those deaths are injection-related. The AIDS death rate for Latinos in this age group is more than double that of whites in the same age group (Day, 1997). Latinos are three times more likely to contract AIDS than to die from an overdose.

Several models are currently being used to address illicit drug use, which, according to statistics, have not been successful.

The Mixed Message Model

When the use of alcohol, tobacco, and prescription, over-the-counter, and illicit drugs are included, almost no one in our society is truly drug-free (Duncan et al., 1994). The "just say no to drugs" model, which declares all drugs bad, has failed to make clear that drugs are neither good nor bad and contradicts the current pervasive drug use in society. Elementary-school age children are confused by this mixed message when they observe treatment for themselves or others with multiple medications. In an effort to discourage illegal drug use, risks and dangers are often exaggerated. Young adults are distrustful because the message is not truthful and causes suspicion regarding information about addiction. Marijuana use may not have made them seek out cocaine or heroin. The typical response of adolescents and young adults to such contradictory information is simply to discredit the message.

The Crime and Punishment Model

The United States spends 65 percent of its drug intervention dollars on incarceration and prosecution, and a mere 35 percent on education, prevention, research, and treatment combined. Theoretically this means if the criminal model was successful, drug use could be reduced by 65 percent. In fact, drug use has steadily increased according to the most current household survey by the National Institute on Drug Abuse (Department of Health and Human Services, 1997).

"Father Knows Best" Model

This disease model prescribes that the intravenous drug user (IDU) must first be detoxified and then taught healthier coping mechanisms. Detoxification can be done either in an inpatient or outpatient program. The length of an inpatient program varies from as little as three days to as long as two months and the availability of beds is limited. An outpatient program can last as long as a year. Approximately 10 percent of the drug-using population enter detoxification programs. The remaining 90 percent includes those who cannot participate because of lack of space and those who do not wish to enter these facilities. Recovery from drug use is not a constant progression. Rather, it involves occasionally falling back a few steps before moving forward again. This model is an all-or-nothing approach that produces more failures than successes.

A new model that has gained interest recently is based on the principle of reducing the risks to both the patient and the community.

The Harm Reduction Model

Harm reduction is a model of care that emerged from the need for an alternative treatment for injection drug users. The theory focuses on maximizing community health interventions that promote safety and reduce drug-related harm. It is a community-based, public health intervention model that provides support and health promotion services to drug users without the requirement that they remain drug-free (Duncan, 1995). This is a radical change from the abstinence-oriented perspective. It requires that one must first accept the inability to control others and respect an individual's choice to use drugs. In using this model of care, the health care professional acknowledges the client's responsibility for his or her own choices. The harm reduction model is based on the following principles:

- All humans have intrinsic value and dignity.
- All have the right to comprehensive nonjudgmental medical and social services.
- Licit and illicit drugs are neither good nor bad.
- Users are competent to make choices.
- Outcomes are in the hands of the patient.
- Options are provided in a nonjudgmental, noncoercive way.

Intrinsic value and dignity are the basis of the professional health care model that is nondiscriminating regardless of the disease. One does not judge a patient with HIV any more or less than one would judge a person with cardiac disease or cancer.

Acknowledging a person's value and dignity is the basis of a trusting relationship that is equally rewarding to both parties. It is the foundation for building the strongest possible positive relationship with a client.

Nonjudgmental medical and social services for comprehensive care of an individual create an atmosphere of caring and concern for the person's well-being. It addresses the whole patient, rather than the drug use issue. Drugs have always been and are likely to remain a part of American culture. Drug use will happen. Instead of becoming morally indignant and punitive, we can assume the existence of drug use and seek to minimize its negative effects (Rosenbaum, 1997).

Users are competent to make choices. Just as any other patient or client, a person who uses drugs is capable of making choices, participating in his or her health care and selecting the best plan of care with the chosen health care provider. Abstinence should never be a criterion for receiving care. The client's and health care professional's goal should be to create a partnership based on appropriate behavior, not sobriety (Lyons, 1996). Outcomes are in the hands of the patient. Assessing and addressing the patients' needs with information, referrals, and options acknowledges their right to determine what results they would like to achieve and what method they would like to employ to gain the results. The responsibility is with the individual.

Although providing options in a nonjudgmental, noncoercive way is a familiar concept in the health care field, it can be difficult to put into practice. Some words set up a hostile, adversarial environment. The terms "noncompliant," "drug seeking," and "difficult" reflect personal judgment by a nurse or social worker. Better terms for describing behaviors would be "nonadherent" or "challenging." The providers' feelings about drug use need to be set aside. The user has a wealth of information that a nonuser needs to learn. The greatest educator on drug use is the patient. Information about illicit drug use, routes of administration, types of drugs used, availability, cost, and methods of payment are a necessary part of the assessment plan. The question, "What can you tell me about heroin use in this area?" will reveal important opportunities for interventions. The plan of care will vary if the drug of choice is heroin, crack, cocaine, or amphetamines. The answers to these questions provide health care professionals with information to suggest ways the client will be able to reduce harm while promoting safety and wellness.

Legal syringe exchange and accessible sterile drug-using and safer-sex equipment are the top priorities in reducing the transmission of the HIV virus. The effectiveness of this harm reduction approach is evident when the statistics from Australia are reviewed. There a needle exchange program has been in place for ten years, and the result has been a reduction in the seroprevalence of HIV among drug users from 50 percent to 2 percent.

Needles and syringes are not designed for reuse. They are difficult to completely clean and disinfect. The only reliable ways to prevent transmission of HIV are to either stop injecting drugs or stop sharing equipment. Needle exchange programs hold promise as an effective intervention to limit HIV transmission.

Despite the fact that access to sterile needles through needle exchange programs has been shown to reduce the transmission of HIV/AIDS among IDUs and their families, there is currently a ban on federal funding for such programs. Only 117 needle exchange programs currently operate in approximately seventy-two cities, relying mainly on volunteers. The ban exists despite seven federally sponsored reports attesting to the efficacy of clean needle exchange for reducing HIV transmission among drug users. Study after study has shown that needle exchange does not lead to an increase in illegal drug use, nor does it lead to new drug users. As an example, a study in Connecticut found that new HIV infections were reduced by 33 percent among needle exchange participants over a year-long period.

Needle exchange programs provide a critical link between IDUs and public health services because workers often refer addicts to treatment programs. A recent study estimated conservatively that from 1987 to 1995 up to 10,000 HIV infections could have been prevented by a national program of needle exchange (Lurie and Drucker, 1997). The cost to the U.S. health care system of treating these preventable cases is an estimated $500 million. The average cost of operating a needle exchange program that can provide services to hundreds is $169,000 a year. The final irony is the comparison between this figure and the average lifetime cost of treating *one* person infected with HIV/AIDS, $119,000.

In 1997 an independent consensus panel convened by the National Institutes of Health found that "an impressive body of evidence suggests powreful effects from needle-exchange programmes . . . there is no longer doubt that these programmes work." Yet, despite this epidemic, the United States remains one of the few industrialised countries that refuses to provide easy access to sterile syringes (Editorial, 1998).

HIV/AIDS is a public health problem without a contemporary parallel. As health care providers become more informed about transmission by intravenous drug use, more and more each year are becoming involved in the prevention and reduction of harm to individuals, families, and communities by volunteering, speaking, and engaging in political actions supporting needle exchange in the United States.

Chapter 1

Give Me the Bottom Line

Hope's physical examination was unremarkable. She was a calm, capable thirty-four-year-old woman with long, sandy-red hair and alabaster skin. She was tall, thin, and well-groomed. She came seeking advice on how to maintain her health shortly after learning she had tested HIV positive. She denied any major physical changes, but did admit to increased frequency of headaches and upper respiratory infections. She also revealed that she believed her risk factor to be injection drug use. She had used heroin intermittently over the past nine years.

Because Hope's immediate concern was coping with her new diagnosis of HIV, the focus of the initial visit was on reducing the stress she was feeling. Her outwardly calm exterior did not reflect her inner chaos.

The Immunology Center is a part of a Northeastern metropolitan hospital. The outpatient setting specializes in patients infected with the HIV virus. A team of health care professionals, infectious disease specialists, obstetrician/gynecologists, nurses, psychologists, nutritionists, and social workers work together to develop care plans based on the individual's need. After introducing themselves, the physician and the nurse asked questions to assess Hope's perception of the meaning of the disease.

When they asked, "How did you hear about this clinic?," she responded, "Two of my best friends are positive. One of my friends has AIDS. She comes to this clinic and likes the way the doctors and nurses treat her." She went on to say that she had decided to get tested knowing her chances of being infected were very high. She had never shared needles with either of these friends, but she had shared needles in the past.

When asked, "What do you know about HIV infection?," she said, "I know it is a disease that I will die from. I just want to live as long as I can."

To assess her personal experience with HIV, the nurse asked, "What is going on with your friend with AIDS?"

Hope described the troublesome symptoms of fatigue, achiness, insomnia, and coughing with which her friend was currently living. She also said she thought the medication that her friend had to take was overwhelming. She couldn't imagine how her friend managed to swallow fourteen pills each day.

In response to the question, "What sorts of changes do you think are ahead for you now?," she said, "I guess I just have to live with it. I got myself into this and now I have to just live with it. I have been around the wrong people for a long time."

Hope was asked about her support network and with whom she could share her diagnosis. "Who are the most important people in your life right now?" She immediately named her seven-year-old daughter, Sarah, as the most important person in her life. Hope's parents were deceased. She had never married and had no significant partner in her life at that time. She had one married sister who lived nearby. Hope said she depended on her two friends for support. They were also both mothers and HIV positive. They all lived in the same neighborhood in the suburbs and spent a lot of time together. Their children played together and the women shared baby-sitting responsibilities. She felt her friends were her support as she was theirs.

After conducting this basic psychosocial assessment, the physician and the nurse went on to assess for signs and symptoms of immune system impairment. The following questions guided Hope's physical assessment:

- How is your appetite? Has your weight changed? Have you had any diarrhea?
- How is your energy level?
- How many hours a day/night do you sleep? Are you rested on awakening?
- How is your vision? Any blurring, spots, or recent changes?
- Have you noticed any changes in your skin? Itchiness, dryness, swelling, irritated, or sore areas?
- Have you experienced any shortness of breath either when resting, walking, or climbing stairs?

• Have you noticed any changes in your throat or mouth? Difficulty swallowing, dryness, or pain?
• How is your memory? Concentration?

Because of the strong association between HIV and abnormal Pap smears and the high incidence of vaginal candida albicans, the following questions were also asked: "Are your menstrual periods regular?" and "Have you noticed any changes in vaginal discharge? Any burning, itching, or pain?"

The physical exam also included an evaluation for symptoms of other sexually transmitted diseases such as gonorrhea, syphilis, venereal warts, hepatitis, and herpes. A Pap smear and two wet mounts were obtained to rule out cervical disease, yeast infection, and trichomoniasis. She was questioned about risks for exposure to tuberculosis. Hope denied having had any of these problems. The questions and examination having been completed, Hope needed basic blood work, including a CD4+ count (often referred to as a T-cell count) as a basis for medical interventions. Hope was asked to return to the clinic in one week so that the results could be discussed and treatments, if necessary, could be reviewed.

The outcome of this initial assessment was that Hope was a candidate for antiretroviral therapy but did not need aggressive prophylaxis because her CD4+ count was over 200. She had some knowledge of HIV infection and expressed a desire for more information. Because she was fatalistic regarding her prognosis and seemed to have low self-esteem, she was at risk for severe depression. She was not identified as a risk for suicide, however, because she had a support network.

Hope was prescribed AZT (zidovudine) three times per day. (Today, she would not have been prescribed monotherapy, as we now know that combination therapy is superior in suppressing viral replication.) She agreed to return to the clinic monthly and as needed for any physical changes or problems. It was explained that regular medical visits, even when a newly diagnosed patient is healthy, are important in order to obtain the best possible outcome for that individual. Because of the risk for depression, she was informed of the availability of both support groups and psychiatric counseling. As expected, she initially declined. However, she was told that these options remained available to her.

The plan of treatment was to assess her general health and immune system monthly. She needed to be screened for tuberculosis and monitored for side effects of the antiretroviral therapy. Our plan of care was to establish trust through unconditional acceptance and caring. She needed education on safety in food preparation, use of bleach solutions for household cleaning, management of menstrual products, and how to practice safer sex. She would also be assessed for weight, sensory, integumentary, gastrointestinal, genitourinary, or neurological changes.

However, had the assessment stopped here, Hope's primary problem would have been missed. Using a harm reduction model meant addressing the concern Hope felt at that moment, which was her new diagnosis. When asked about current drug use, she denied that she was currently using. She told of her struggles with detoxification, admitting to participation in treatment programs eight times over the past nine years. Each time she had been unable to stay straight. Alcohol use was also a key problem and she agreed that alcohol had often led the way back to her intravenous drug use.

A diagnosis of HIV infection compounds daily stress for an IDU. Many IDUs feel they deserve to be infected. Society condemns IDUs with the attitude that "they get everything they deserve, including HIV." Guilt about being infected is as devastating as the fear of the disease. Hope was assured that regardless of the route of transmission, no one deserves this disease. Of primary importance, however, was the need to establish a trust relationship in order to allow her to look at her primary problem: recurrent IV drug use. The issue of relapse prevention was addressed each visit in some way.

Because relapse often occurs, anticipating it can assist in developing a plan of care. Ask the following questions:

- What have been triggers for you in the past when you have relapsed?
- Do certain friends or places remind you of when you have used in the past?
- How did you avoid drugs during the times you were clean?
- How do you deal with stressful situations?

- Are you attending support groups, such as Narcotics Anonymous? Have you in the past?
- In what ways can we support you to prevent you from relapsing?
- How many alcoholic drinks have you had in the last week?

Hope followed the recommendations for monthly clinic visits for the next two years. During that time she did undergo disease progression. On one clinic visit she had a low-grade fever. She also had had a five-pound weight loss since her previous visit three weeks earlier. She complained of loss of appetite, not being able to taste her food, and difficulty swallowing. An examination of her throat revealed white patches on the soft palate and the posterior lingual area. She was diagnosed with oral candida albicans (also known as thrush). Although the esophagus could not be examined easily, her symptoms were consistent with esophagitis, which could also be caused by the same fungal infection. The treatment prescribed was fluconazole 100 mg daily for seven days along with a lidocaine spray to relieve the pain.

On the fifth day after starting this therapy, Hope was called and she reported feeling much better. Her appetite had also returned. On another occasion Hope presented with a fever of 101° F, a cough and shortness of breath when walking even short distances. She also admitted that she had relapsed and had been using heroin for the past few days. She was assessed for possible complications of IV drug use, such as cellulitis and endocarditis, as well as bacterial pneumonia and *pneumocystis carinii* pneumonia (PCP). Her chest X ray showed a left lower lobe infiltrate. A sputum sample for culture and sensitivity was obtained prior to antibiotic therapy. She was diagnosed with bacterial pneumonia and treated successfully with an oral antibiotic. Otherwise, she had no complications from the HIV disease over these years.

The importance of regular medical visits, even when a newly diagnosed patient is healthy, is to obtain the best outcome possible for that individual. They are, over time, the way to establish trust through unconditional acceptance and caring. Trust depends on that individual's past experiences as well as those of the health care professional.

Repeatedly, Hope expressed her concern for her daughter. She said that she knew her chances of "being around" until her daughter reached adulthood were slim. Hope's diagnosis with HIV was her wake-up call. She was reevaluating her life. These realizations were unfolding during her regular appointments.

Hope came into clinic one day and asked for help with her IV drug use problem. She was ready. She did not want a simple five-to-seven-day inpatient detoxification program. She was ready for a longer inpatient program. This would not only clear her system of drugs, but also help her to learn alternative coping skills for stressful situations through counseling and support group meetings.

Knowing that her commitment might waver created urgency for placement in a detoxification program as soon as possible. The policy must be to "strike while the iron is hot." Hope had mustered all her strength to ask for help. This was a difficult, life-changing decision. Any delay could mean that she would go back into the environment where people, places, and situations become triggers that lead to drug use.

Hope wanted to enter the program the next day. This was a cause for concern because she might change her mind overnight. However, she adamantly promised that she would follow through after making arrangements for her daughter. Because the relationship between Hope and the team was ongoing and positive, it was believed that she would follow through. The second obstacle was Hope's family. Her sister, Ann, had been through this before. She had taken care of Sarah each of the many times Hope had gone into a short-term detoxification program. She had watched Hope fail each time. Ann was as adamant as Hope that this would, indeed, be the last time she would look after Sarah.

Hope did succeed. This time was the right time. When asked about her experience in the rehabilitation program, she said it was the best thing that ever happened to her.

A short four months later, Hope developed cytomegalovirus (CMV) retinitis. This opportunistic infection is very serious because it can lead to blindness. Although new therapies are now available, at that time the treatment was lifelong intravenous therapy. Therefore, it required a surgically implanted central venous access for daily drug delivery. Hope had a Hickman catheter placed and was referred to a home care/home infusion company for instruction in medication setup and administration as well as home support.

Referring a patient to a home care agency can be very depressing for the patient. It is seen as a milestone in the progression of the disease. Therefore, it is important to discuss the implications of the services, their benefits, and to sprinkle the referral generously with hope. Hope needed help immediately with training in home infusions and catheter care. It was explained to her that if she felt comfortable and the clinic felt she was safe, the home care services could be discontinued after the home training was complete.

Hope never discharged herself from the home care agency. Over time the social worker from the agency worked diligently with Hope addressing the tough questions: custody of her daughter, power of attorney, and advance directives. The questions were resolved and Hope developed a new coping system.

Hope was now attending clinic on a weekly basis. Her CD4+ count was 100 and she was diagnosed with AIDS. Because of her susceptibility to opportunistic infections, Hope was given prophylactic therapy. Her new regime was Bactrim DS (TMP/SMX [trimethoprim/sulphamethoxazole]) one daily to prevent PCP, fluconazole 100 mg three times a week to prevent fungal infections, and continuing the AZT. She was continually reassessed for changes in vision, indicating a progression of the CMV retinitis, fever, cough, or shortness of breath, weight loss, vomiting, or diarrhea, skin lesions or ulcerations, burning, tingling in her extremities, changes in memory or concentration, and dizziness or an unsteady gait. Her psychosocial status was evaluated through questions such as:

- How are things going at home?
- Are you sleeping at night?
- How often have you cried during the past week?
- Do you feel proud of the fact that you have remained drug-free for the last few months?

During one medical appointment several months after beginning the home IV therapy, Hope was asked about her relationship with Sarah. Hope disclosed that they were having problems. Hope had to hide her Hickman catheter. Her dressing changes and infusions had to be done when Sarah was not at home. Sarah was very angry much of the time, and she became even angrier whenever she saw Hope's catheter or treatments. Their small family had undergone major changes. Because of Hope's recovery from drug use, Sarah, now nine years old, had gained a full-time mom. Sarah had also seen her mother's best friend recently die of AIDS. She was being confronted with changes because of her mother's illness. Sarah's anger was her coping mechanism for survival. It was clear that a nine-year-old would have to struggle to hide the pure terror she must be feeling.

Hope and Sarah were referred to a community agency that provided case management for families affected by the AIDS virus. The case manager arranged for family and individual counseling.

Several months again went by before the medical staff received a call from Hope's sister, Ann. She was at Hope's home. She had discovered Hope lying on the couch, where she had been for several days. Ann said Hope had been neglecting her daughter and sounded "nuts." The home care agency arranged for transportation for Hope to come to the medical center for evaluation. She was diagnosed with bacterial pneumonia and admitted to the hospital.

Hope's change in mental status was due to hypoxemia and fever. Although the pneumonia and confusion were cleared with standard medical interventions, it was apparent that Hope was no longer able to care for herself, let alone Sarah. Ann also believed it was no longer safe for Sarah to live with Hope and had taken her into her own home. The physician, nurse, community agency social worker, and Ann met with Hope to decide on the best way to deal with the situation. Hope was keenly aware of her limitations. She also wanted to do the right thing by her daughter. She decided that it would be best for her to go to a nursing home.

Because of the particular community, an alternative for Hope was a group home for people with AIDS. This home was staffed by a nurse during the day and home health aide for twenty-four hours. After visiting the facility with her family, Hope chose to live there. This allowed her as much independence as possible and the joy of having Sarah visit for the weekends.

Hope had previously arranged for Ann to have not only legal custody of Sarah, but also legal power of attorney and durable power of attorney. This would allow Ann to act on her behalf if she were unable to express her desires. Hope wanted no life support measures should she be hospitalized in the future.

During the three and a half years that Hope was followed by the team at the medical center, she inspired many health care professionals with her grace and dignity. The challenge faced by this team was to look beneath her cool, easygoing manner at the deeper, root issue of IV drug use. With support and encouragement, she overcame an addiction and faced the toughest of all journeys, leaving all who worked with her in awe.

LESSON 1: ASSESSMENT OF PRIMARY PROBLEMS

Recognizing and prioritizing problems is vital to effective treatment. The patient with a dual diagnosis may actually have a triple or quadruple diagnosis. It is not unusual for mental illness or psychosocial trauma to compete with addiction and HIV-positive status as the first problem to be addressed.

Because of the complexity of physical, mental, and psychosocial problems, setting up the plan of treatment and plan of care for the management of the patient with a dual diagnosis presents a tremendous challenge. Each professional discipline has standardized terminology for identifying these problems. The process involves developing a plan of action and a plan of evaluation based on the initial assessment. The physician's assessment will lead to establishing medical diagnoses based on the findings of the physical examination, the history given on interview, and the results of laboratory and radiology testing. Because the goal of medical care is to treat illness, this assessment is used to develop the plan of treatment.

The nurse's assessment will also involve recording subjective and objective information regarding past and current health issues. The nursing diagnoses are based on actual or potential alterations in health status. As in all areas of nursing, the goals are to promote wellness, to treat human responses to illness, and to identify the patient's need for education and follow-up. The nursing assessment is used to develop the plan of care.

The social worker's assessment will identify past and present psychosocial needs as well as a pattern of high-risk behavior. The social worker's plan of care will determine interventions needed to promote safety and provide psychosocial support.

A Midwestern team of AIDS specialists concluded that "Chemical dependency in a setting of HIV disease is frequently the primary diagnosis, which, if not addressed initially, will sabotage any further medical interventions geared to management of the HIV disease itself" (Snyder, Kaempfer, and Ries, 1996, p. 74).

Developing a comprehensive plan of treatment and an effective plan of care begins with understanding the drug history and the current use. The process is the same as for any assessment: develop objectives, set goals, and evaluate outcomes. The difference may be in the type of interview and the questions asked.

Sometimes obtaining correct information is a matter of knowing whom to ask. Chances are, the chemically dependent, HIV-positive patient seeking medical care has been involved with other community services. Behaviors can reveal certain mental health disorders. On the other hand, substance use can cause mood changes and personality changes that mimic organic disorders. Ask for the names of individuals or agencies with whom the patient has worked well in the past. Dates of service from community agencies or previous physicians will corroborate a vague history. All inconsistencies need verification from pharmacies, case managers, or family members. Ask questions such as:

- What services have you used in the past?
- How did they help you?
- How did you hear about those services?
- How often do you use them?
- When do you return?
- How did you hear about us?

Sometimes asking the right questions will obtain the needed answers. Having a standard opening line, such as "What's been going on with you lately?," will invite comments about the patient's general sense of well-being and state of mind. Asking "Why are you here this morning?" will focus the answer on events that occurred immediately before to either making the appointment or showing up in the clinic. Phrase questions to elicit explanations rather than yes or no answers. Explore the psychosocial history carefully. Respond respectfully to the answers.

Ask directly about what drugs the patient has used in the past and when was the last time they were used. This is an opportunity to assess high-risk behaviors and apply the harm reduction principles. The answer to any question is important in developing a total picture of the patient. Ask questions such as:

- What drugs do you use?
- How do you use them?
- Do you smoke, snort, swallow, inhale, or inject?

- Where do you inject (muscle, vein, or skin pop)?
- Where do you use (home, other's home, shooting gallery)?
- How often do you use (daily, weekly, in binges)?
- When was the last time?
- Where do you get your needles?
- Do you have a needle exchange in your community?
- Do you share needles with anyone?
- How do you dispose of your needles?
- Have you ever been in a detoxification program?
- What is the longest time you have been drug-free?
- Are you on a methadone maintenance program?
- How do you support your habit?
- Have you ever had a drug-related health problem (e.g., cellulitis, endocarditis, septicemia, cotton fever)?

Sometimes it is a matter of how the questions are asked. If the diagnosis of HIV/AIDS was made several years before, the patient may be familiar with the questions routinely asked by a health practitioner thus anticipating the answers that the practitioner expects and wants to hear. It is important to establish that the only expectation is that the patient will be honest and open. If the practitioner displays empathy, the patient will be more likely to share symptoms honestly. On the other hand, if the practitioner is tense and rushed, the patient will also give a shortened version or incomplete answers. Being judgmental about a patient's choice of living style or drug use will greatly reduce the chances of establishing an open relationship. Suggestions for creating a relaxed environment:

- Smile.
- Use physical touch.
- Make eye contact.
- Speak clearly.
- Pay attention to your body language and any messages sent by your facial expressions.
- Know the signs and symptoms of psychiatric disorders as well as physical diseases.
- Express appreciation for the patient's honesty in sharing his or her story with you.

If you do not understand the street drug terminology used, ask the patient. The patient will usually be happy to educate the health care provider. Assuming rather than clarifying can lead to distrust. It also depicts a lack of interest in what is being said. In turn, the education the health care provider intends to share will be more readily accepted.

Obtaining accurate information is a process that requires a commitment to holistic care. The patient with HIV disease usually is followed by one physician or clinic for all health care needs. Because of this, the responsibility for comprehensive care and follow-up falls on that individual or team.

The responsibility for establishing a plan of treatment rests with this primary team. The success or failure of that plan depends on two things. The first is the accuracy of problem identification. The second is how well the interventions are carried out.

Chapter 2

The Sky Is Not the Limit

Miguel had been around the block so many times he could pace himself to make all the green lights. Miguel knew who to call, at what time of day, when each month, and which individual within the agency to ask for a certain service. Miguel's strong Hispanic accent could be misleading. He had lived in the northeastern United States for twenty-five years. Despite the fact that he spoke, read, and understood English very well, he frequently apologized when asking questions, saying that he was "trying to learn the language." His shy, yet gracious manners and impeccable grooming invited nurturing. At the time Miguel first came to the clinic, he was forty-one years old. He had recently left prison, where he had served a two-year sentence for robbery.

He was born in Puerto Rico and moved to the northeastern United States where he finished high school and one year of college. He left college to work full-time and marry the woman he had been dating for three years. A year later he became a father. Miguel described experimenting with marijuana and pills as a teenager, but he did not begin IV drug use until age twenty-one. His drug use and related problems escalated and five years later, he and his wife divorced. However, Miguel kept in close contact with his wife and daughter, remembering holidays and birthdays. This was a challenge for him because maintaining his heroin habit required most of his time and all of his energy, when he was not in and out of jail. Any stabilizing influence he had came from his mother and his sister. Although his address was the same as theirs, he felt most at home on the streets.

Miguel was diagnosed HIV positive while in prison. He was released on five years' parole and was referred to both a parole office and a program for HIV-positive individuals to facilitate integration into the community. He began coming to the clinic on a regular monthly basis. Because his CD4+ count was close to 300, he accepted the option of antiretroviral therapy. He had no other medical problems at this time other than recurring sinusitis and headaches. He qualified for disability and was required to designate a person to act as a payee for his monthly checks. He named his sister as his payee.

Within a few months, however, he had relapsed into cocaine and heroin use. His counselor through the integration program advocated for him and prevented him from being sent back to prison. Instead, he enrolled in a methadone program. He was able to adhere to the program rules and avoid relapse into IV drug use completely throughout the next seven years. He did have periodic cocaine use and frequently swapped tranquilizers with others.

He continued to be followed medically. His CD4+ count dropped to 152 following an episode of sepsis secondary to sinusitis and pneumonia. He began prophylaxis with Bactrim (TMP/SMX) and a second antiretroviral. He was also on cimetidine and a bronchodialating inhaler. While hospitalized, he began Xanax (alprazolam) for anxiety. For three years, his CD4+ count remained between 140 and 180. He tolerated these prescriptions and kept his clinic appointments. Periods of weight loss and worsening of headaches could consistently be related to increased time spent on the streets and to exposure to both harsh weather and cocaine use.

Miguel did not like to get up too early in the morning. The methadone program was open for dosing between 6:00 a.m. and 10:00 a.m. This was a time problem because, although the program was only about five miles from his home, he had to take two buses to get there. This was also a financial problem. Being on disability entitled him to ride the bus free before 8:00 a.m. and between the hours of 10:00 a.m. and 3:00 p.m. While he was committed to the daily routine, he did not succeed at catching a bus early enough to get him back home by 8:00 a.m. Neither did he like the option of staying at the program center until 10:00 a.m. Miguel's solution was to rotate calling each HIV/AIDS organization for bus passes. After doing this for about a year, each agency began to recognize the pattern and refused to issue them. One day Miguel came into clinic very upset about "the way I am being treated." He said, "I am supposed to be able to get help from these people. I need help because I have HIV." Although Miguel was obviously an intelligent person, no amount of explaining the limits of the system made sense to him.

Another routine request Miguel made was for food vouchers. After several months of filling requests on a regular basis, his social worker felt the need to explore the reasons why he repeatedly ran out of food. Obviously, there was something more complicated going on. The approach of handing out a voucher was only a short-term solution. It was known that he lived with his mother at that point, and reports from the community were that she was a caring person and a good homemaker. It was also known that his sister, as payee, was involved in his life and concerned about his welfare.

The clinic social worker made an appointment with him to discuss the situation openly and honestly. She began the session with, "Here is the situation. You have needed to ask for food vouchers three times over the last two months. I don't recall you ever doing that before. What is different recently?"

He answered, "Nothing is different. I just thought I could get a food voucher sometimes."

The social worker answered, "These services are certainly available and you are entitled as much as anyone else. My concern is that you have not needed them in the past, yet recently you do."

Miguel said, "I just don't have any money to buy food. I only get what my sister gives me."

The social worker said, "I understand that, Miguel, but do you agree that this is a change for you?"

"Yes," he said, "my mother usually takes care of the cooking. She went to visit my brother in Puerto Rico last month. She is not home to cook for me."

"Miguel, did you ask your sister for money for food?"

"Yes, I did. She brings me groceries and then she thinks that is all I need. But I need other things sometimes."

"I see several choices here. You could ask her to buy those special things or you could ask her for the money and do the shopping yourself."

"The problem is that my brothers and nieces and nephews come over and eat all my food. And once in awhile I have a friend over for dinner. I will talk to my sister about it and I will make a list and ask her to buy the things that I want."

"Okay. Are you interested in the cooking classes that are going to begin next week? You might learn a new recipe."

"Actually, I am getting tired of ham and cheese sandwiches. I would like to go."

When Miguel's mother returned from Puerto Rico, they found that during their separation they had gotten used to living alone. Miguel found an apartment within walking distance from his mother's house so he could visit often. This created a new financial challenge for Miguel and the social worker. After several months he came to ask for rental assistance.

"I need $100 to pay my rent next week. I have to pay it on time or the landlord says he will not let me stay."

"Okay, Miguel, it is very important to us that you have a safe place to live. We don't want you to be evicted."

"That's good! I was afraid to ask for the money."

"Well, we need to look at why you are short this month. Let's go over your expenses."

"I don't understand why you can't just give me the money. Aren't you supposed to help people?"

"We certainly are. And we can help you even more if we can prevent you from being short *next* month as well. We have a rule that we give money for any sort of assistance once a year. If we give you this money now, we won't be able to give you money again for rent, heat, or the telephone until next year. It is important to us that we know we are doing what is the best for you."

"Well, maybe I better ask my sister for the money this time. I spent my rent money on Christmas presents and I think she will give it back to me. I may need money another time."

Once settled into the routine of living alone, Miguel found he enjoyed the freedom of living alone with few commitments. He became involved in the local drop-in center for PLW (persons living with) HIV/AIDS. He began attending a support group for Hispanic IDUs at the methadone program and initiated the formation of a support group for Hispanic men with HIV and IV drug use. These activities meant he was seldom home. This was a problem for the counselor from the prison transition program, who was required to make a weekly home visit. The support she provided kept many HIV-positive clients out of jail. She made herself accessible by sharing her beeper number with her clients. She would phone clients the day before to remind them of appointments. She faithfully kept her appointments with her clients. All of her clients, including Miguel, cared about and respected her as a person. Therefore, it was always mysterious why Miguel would often not be home for their appointments.

She would ask, "Miguel, where were you today? I waited fifteen minutes and you did not come home."

He would smile and say, "Oh, I was on my way. You should have waited for me. I was home just a few minutes after you left.

"You know, Miguel, I have a beeper. All you have to do is call me and say you are going to be late. This is the polite way of changing an appointment."

"I know. I am sorry. Listen, how about if you meet me at the coffee shop downtown?"

"No, I can't do that. The rules are that I see you in your home. I need to know that you are living in a safe place."

"Okay. I will be at home next week."

"The next time this happens, I will have to report it to the parole officer."

"No, no, please don't do that. I promise, I will remember to keep my appointments with you!"

Miguel would also test the limits of the case manager, whose role was to provide transportation on an as-needed basis for mandatory appointments. He called the clinic one day to say that he was at the local HIV/AIDS chapter. He had come there by bus, directly from the methadone program. He now was feeling ill and needed to go home. The case manager knew him well and knew that he had indeed been ill at times in the past. On arrival, however, Miguel walked out of the building, greeted the case manager with a smile, and jumped into the car. Under his arm was a case of nutritional supplements. When asked about feeling ill, Miguel replied that he felt a lot better now. The case manager suspected that Miguel had called simply to avoid having to travel by bus carrying the heavy case. He decided to confront Miguel frankly and politely with his suspicion.

Miguel confirmed that he had not been telling the truth about feeling ill. The case manager reviewed the rules for transportation and explained why the clinic had to set limits on when and where rides were given. Miguel was not pleased by these limitations but agreed to follow the rules.

Miguel was involved in a barter system within his neighborhood. People traded certain prescribed medications. Miguel had been on Xanax for seven years by now. One morning he walked into the clinic pale, diaphoretic, and shaking. His pulse, blood pressure, and temperature were elevated. He refused to go to the emergency room. He knew that it was too early to get his Xanax refilled, but he wondered if the doctor could make an exception. Miguel had come in the previous month requesting that his Xanax be changed from twice to three times a day. He claimed adamantly that he needed a midday dose to discipline himself to stay home in the afternoons and avoid going out with friends who used cocaine. He also needed the early morning and nighttime doses to manage his anxiety. He was now presenting with acute symptoms of withdrawal. It was apparent that he had been unable to discipline himself enough to avoid overuse or trading. In order to safely promote his independence, Miguel was given a prescription for weekly refills and referred to his methadone counselor for support.

Miguel continues to thrive in the community. Being functionally independent is an important factor in his community involvement. It would be a disservice to create dependency for financial assistance, transportation, or early refills. By promoting his independence, his support team encourages him to learn to anticipate his own needs and solve his own problems. With these skills, he can change his own expectations for success.

LESSON 2: SETTING BEHAVIORAL LIMITS

To fulfill the responsibilities of an HIV/AIDS provider, a practitioner must understand the standards of the profession. In order to gain the respect of the patient, the team, and the community, the health care worker must understand the expectations of the employer/agency.

Team members must be committed to the team's overall plan of care to focus on the best interest of the patient. By evaluating the outcome of the interventions at regular team meetings, the plan can be continued or altered. It may be helpful for the new team member to focus on the fact that he or she is a representative of and responsible to the policies of the organization. Team members should adhere to policies. If one member is offering services not ordinarily provided (such as rides, food, food vouchers, equipment, clothing, or after-hours support) the community will perceive that other team members are not doing their job.

Team meetings should provide an opportunity for members to learn from each other. There should be discussion about perceived errors in judgment. Rumors or knowledge about mistakes should be validated. Effective interventions should be shared and successes should be acknowledged.

The goals of the health care team for the HIV-positive substance user are based on physical and psychosocial needs, functional status, and available support systems. A practitioner has no control over whether a patient actually follows a plan of care. When deciding short-term goals, the patient should always be involved. A patient has a right to (1) accept, (2) refuse, or (3) demand available treatment. On the other hand, the professional health care worker has a responsibility to determine if a plan of care is appropriate and likely to succeed. Some examples of ineffective care planning are:

- providing written materials to someone who cannot read;
- considering supplies and equipment for the homeless; and
- recommending complex medication regimes for someone with dementia.

Being available for visits is a criterion for remaining in service. To encourage compliance with a visit schedule, the home health care worker sends the message that the individual is valued. This can be done through repeated, unconditional, nonjudgmental contact either in person or by telephone.

The process of behavior change should be looked at as a long-term goal. One model of behavior change is the Transtheoretical Model of Change (Prochaska et al., 1994). This model identifies five stages of self-awareness that every individual must progress through before change can happen. These stages are precontemplative, contemplative, preparation, action, and maintenance.

In the precontemplative stage, the individual is unaware of the problem. The health care worker can plant the seed of the idea that change is an option to consider in the future. In the contemplative stage, the individual is aware of and considering the need for change. Secondary prevention is appropriate at this time. This involves appropriate early intervention and education following the identification of a primary problem.

In the preparation stage, the individual needs direction as well as support to plan for and successfully make that change. In the action stage, the individual has stopped the undesirable behavior. The health care worker needs to be prepared to present ways to manage frustrations that will arise. Finally, in the maintenance stage, the individual will need the unconditional trust and support of the health care team to succeed at permanently changing a lifestyle. It may be appropriate to remind individuals of the disadvantages and hardships of the lifestyle of active drug use. A new support network may have to be built. Should the individual relapse, it is important for the health care team to continue to help the individual rise above the guilt associated with failure and to try again.

If home visits are either unaccepted or unsafe, telephone contact can ensure that the patient is not completely lost to the health care system. Friendly, consistent contact will assure the patient that resources are available when he or she is ready to take advantage of them. This is meeting the patient at his or her own level of need. Respecting the patient's right to make choices will promote a sense of self-esteem and encourage positive, health-promoting behaviors.

Chapter 3

So, What's the Point?

While it could be presumed that April's aunt intended to ensure that April used only clean needles, the fact that she, too, was an active IV drug user complicated the issue. It is not uncommon for drug use to be a family issue. April and her aunt, who was an insulin-dependent diabetic, had both been using heroin for about five years before their world collapsed.

At twenty-nine, April was released from prison following a two-year sentence. Because she had been diagnosed HIV positive during her incarceration, she was referred to the outpatient infectious disease clinic for follow-up.

On her initial clinic visit, a complete drug history was conducted. She shared that although she had been clean during her prison stay, she was now using five bags of heroin a day. April had intended to remain drug-free upon her release but found herself back in the same environment, with the same friends. A bag of heroin in the current market was anywhere from $7 to $10, so she needed $35 to $50 per day just to support her current use. She supported her habit by working the streets as a prostitute.

Her number one priority was finding a safe place to live. Her apartment was in an inner-city, socioeconomically deprived area, amid much drug use and violence.

There were several concerns regarding April's current lifestyle and injection practices. She stated that she did not share needles, but usually disposed of them in the trash.

Alternative disposal methods were discussed: (a) a safer method would be putting them in a can with a lid (such as a coffee can) or (b) taking needles to a needle exchange, where dirty needles are replaced by clean ones. A second concern was that April often shared injection equipment, such as cookers and filters, with her friends.

When asked if she had ever been through a detoxification program, April stated that she had been in a five-day detoxification program twice, and a thirty-day program once. April agreed the latter was the most successful, as she had remained drug-free for the following eighteen months. When the nurse offered to make a referral to a program, April said it was not the right time. She was more concerned about other problems. She was also adamant that a methadone maintenance program was not an option. She knew friends who had found that trying to get off methadone was worse than trying to get off heroin.

She had been hospitalized once for cellulitis in her left arm secondary to an infected injection site, which required treatment with intravenous antibiotics. April volunteered that she had had "cotton fever" several times in the past. She expressed her resignation to these complications when she said, "that happens when you shoot up." Cotton fever is a term used for symptoms that manifest as trembling, sweating, headache, and fever. Symptoms are identical to those of a serious bacterial infection such as sepsis or endocarditis. It is believed by drug users to be caused by the cotton filter through which the liquid drug passes in order to remove undissolved particles. Many times the filter is a used cigarette filter. The contaminants can come from the filter, the water used to dilute the drug, used injection equipment, or from other substances mixed with the drug.

As a result of this initial assessment, several areas of concern were identified. These were first brought up by April during the interview process, and then restated by the nurse in a clear, simple manner. April was then asked to verify that they were areas of concern and to clarify their order of importance. At this point, a mutually agreed-upon plan was easily developed and the above goals were the guide. Interventions included referral, education, safer injecting techniques, safer sex, and safer drug use.

April was referred to a local case management agency for housing assistance. A signed release was obtained enabling communication about April's case between agencies. The nurse made the initial call referring her. April was responsible for keeping the appointment with the agency. She eventually did contact the case management agency and relocated to a safer part of town, but she was well aware that reducing drug use was more complicated than changing her environmental circumstances.

Because April might not always have access to her aunt's insulin syringes, she needed information about the local needle exchange program: its hours of operation and location, the fact that clean needles could be obtained on a one-for-one basis (one clean needle for one dirty needle), and that it also supplied bleach, cotton balls (for filters), cookers, and alcohol wipes.

Further, it was explained that whatever contaminants are on the skin at the injection site are put into the bloodstream. Because the normal skin bacteria include microorganisms and viruses, local infection or sepsis may occur. This can be avoided by using alcohol wipes prior to injecting. April was asked to demonstrate how she might use an alcohol wipe. Disconcerted, April began to rub in a back-and-forth motion on her arm. The nurse explained that this motion simply moved the bacteria around. She was congratulated, however, because she seemed to be aware of the practice of harm reduction. The better way of cleansing the skin, by wiping once in one direction only at the site of injection, was demonstrated.

April said that she used condoms most of the time but had been unable to approach the subject with a couple of regular clients. She wasn't sure she could, she said, without disclosing her HIV-positive status. The nurse suggested that April use the fact that these clients knew that she had other sexual partners to discuss how condom use would prevent the inadvertent transmission of sexually transmitted diseases (STDs) from one to the other. April agreed to try this approach because she knew this was a way for her to prevent transmitting the HIV without admitting her personal status.

April expressed that she would like to gradually reduce the amount of heroin she used to avoid symptoms of withdrawal, which could cause relapse. She thought she would start by using four bags a day for the next month. In the meantime, she would limit contact with other people, actively keeping to a prescribed regimen of diet, exercise, and medication.

As April had no health problems related to her HIV and required no new antiretrovirals or prophylaxis, her living arrangements and drug use were the key to establishing a positive relationship based on respect, trust, and confidentiality.

To evaluate the effectiveness of the care plan, April agreed to visit the clinic on a weekly basis. This would enable close contact and support. It also would facilitate the development of mutual trust and respect. Over the next few months, April was not always able to meet her personal goal of gradually reducing her drug use, but she was able to trust the health care team enough to admit freely when relapses occurred. Positive reinforcement was given for the times she did reduce her drug use, and encouragement during the times she was unable to reach her goal.

It takes time to replace old coping mechanisms with new ones, and it almost always requires a tremendous support system during the transition. Hard work and a positive attitude by the health care professional can enable a successful transition over time. Patience and perseverance are required to complete the necessary initial assessment and follow-up. April's story is ongoing; the end has not yet been written. She remains an example of the fortitude and tenacity needed to overcome addiction.

LESSON 3: APPLYING THE HARM REDUCTION MODEL

Harm reduction is the underlying theme in developing a plan of care for the active IV drug user. The goal is to agree first on priorities and then on the means to meet these goals:

1. safe housing;
2. education to reduce harmful lifestyle practices;
3. education to increase personal safety through reducing infection (cellulitis and cotton fever), safer injecting techniques, and safer working practices; and
4. detoxification options; a plan to reduce drug use.

Case management agencies are invaluable in providing guidance to patients who are sincere in their desire to find safe housing by supplying information about available government subsidies, cooperative landlords, and group housing. The availability of local needle exchange programs, hours of operation, and location are necessary for supporting safer injection practice.

Most IV drug users are unaware of the extent of exposure to potential infection through dirty equipment. Because contaminants are present in used cigarette filters, the use of cotton balls should be encouraged. In addition, a new filter should be used every time. Cookers (usually metal bottle caps in which the drug is dissolved) are also a source of contamination. A new cooker should be used each time. Since tap water is also another contaminated substance, using sterile water is recommended. Patients should be reminded to never borrow, share, or lend cookers, filters, or water.

Condoms are essential for commercial sex workers. The expense is a problem. Free condoms (male and female) are usually available at the local needle exchange program as well as other community agencies. It is helpful to be able to give specific information about the location of these agencies to encourage condom use.

When narcotic drugs are taken habitually, a tolerance is developed. As use continues, the tolerance increases. Physical addiction occurs when the body continually needs higher doses to maintain the ability to perform ordinary daily functions without experiencing strong cravings. At this time it is very difficult to stop or even cut down without experiencing discomfort. Withdrawal symptoms are both physical and emotional. The physical symptoms are clammy skin, uncontrolled yawning, runny nose and tears, diarrhea, sweating, vomiting, stomach and leg cramps, and disturbed sleep. Withdrawal from alcohol and pills also includes hallucinations and seizures. Emotional symptoms include extreme craving and mood swings, irritability, euphoria, fear, panic attacks, depression, suicidal thoughts, hopelessness, and a sense of isolation. To address the patient holistically, it is important to use every opportunity for the presentation of information in a consistent and timely manner.

Chapter 4

Flattery Will Get You Nowhere

On the clinic wall hangs a plaque that reads, "Please pick your excuse by number." The list begins with "I forgot" and covers the range of reasons for not accomplishing what was expected. Included are mechanical failures, as of alarm clocks and automobiles, unreliable helpers such as spouses and neighbors, accidents, and acts of God such as fire or flood. Jerry could always come up with one more. The bottom line was that he could keep you laughing all the way to the emergency room. In reality, though, Jerry was not in the least bit funny. In fact, he was a sad, neglected, and unresourceful IV drug user.

Jerry's strength was in salesmanship. He could have convinced an Eskimo to buy ice. If the home care worker found him home alone, he would invent friends to prove his popularity. Being a prostitute, he was occasionally found with a client. Rather than reveal the actual relationship, he would create a story about that poor soul's lonely and destitute state requiring Jerry's help. Despite the fact that he was an only child, he spoke at length about his nieces' and nephews' misfortunes. Although he was often homeless, he could hold one's attention for hours as he described his ongoing, simultaneous careers as an engineer, a security guard, and a decorator.

Jerry said he was diagnosed as HIV positive six years before at age twenty-four. At 5'8" and 130 pounds, he presented to the clinic in generally good health, stating he had only been hospitalized once for "food poisoning." He had been hopping from one clinic to another since then. He admitted that as long as he felt strong and well most of the time, he ignored his health care needs. Recently he had been increasingly tired and uncomfortable, and had lost about ten pounds. Also, he said, he was concerned about increasing hair loss. While this was not obvious to others, he was worried about premature baldness. He had been working at various jobs, easily supporting himself "and his family." Although he had finished high school, his subsequent education had been "on-the-job training." Although he denied having any risk factors for HIV related to either IV drug use or sexual activity, he admitted he knew that the virus was limited to transmission by these routes.

On Jerry's second clinic visit he was informed that his CD4+ count had fallen to 125, signifying that the HIV had progressed to AIDS. In addition, his liver enzymes were significantly elevated. When he received this information, he became very quiet for a few moments. While briefly shaken up, however, he seemed to assess the situation and then asked, "I'll be able to get the top-of-the-line pain medication now, right?"

Although Jerry was referred for immediate counseling to help him deal with this news about his health, he chose to leave the clinic. When he did not make an appointment for follow-up, it was believed he would, unfortunately, next be seen in the hospital with a complication of AIDS. Instead, he came as a walk-in several weeks later asking for advice on managing hair loss and requesting something for pain. In his special, charming way he complimented each staff member on some aspect of their appearance or performance. He was started on three medications during this visit: Bactrim (TMP/SMX) for PCP prophylaxis, AZT (zidovudine) as an initial antiretroviral, and a nonsteroidal anti-inflammatory drug (NSAID) for generalized discomfort. He was given an appointment for nutritional consultation and a follow-up clinic visit and was strongly urged to consider alcohol/substance use counseling as indicated by the potential liver damage. He left with a food voucher and a list of local AIDS service agencies. While he did return to clinic a month or so later, he did not follow up on either the nutritionist or the counseling.

Over the next several months, Jerry's clinic visits were erratic. Invariably he made a point of complimenting the examining nurse and physician on their professionalism and compassion on each and every visit. Although it was recommended that he follow the prescribed prophylaxis regime, it was clear that he was not refilling his prescriptions. He reported increasing disabling pain in both feet, his lower legs, and lower back. He began a pain management regime of Vicodin (hydrocodone) with the NSAID as an adjunctive. When this seemed ineffective, he was prescribed Elavil 25 mg at bedtime. His tales of worldly success and interpersonal relationships and support did not coincide with his appearance, which was slightly disheveled and unorganized, nor with his routine appeals for food vouchers.

Eventually, on one clinic visit, Jerry appeared visibly short of breath and his gait had developed a limp. His blood work reflected worsening liver function. He could not recall the last time he had taken any of his medication other than the Vicodin prescribed for peripheral neuropathy. His CD4+ count had dropped below 50.

Although he usually presented as pleasant and cheerful despite obvious hardships, there was one occasion on which Jerry revealed a side of his personality yet unseen. Jerry greeted the receptionist with a single nod. He sat down apart from the other patients and did not speak to anyone. When his name was called, he jumped up and hurried into the examining room. He spoke harshly about the amount of time he had had to wait. He stated loudly that he was entitled to see the doctor of his choice, not whomever happened to be available. As he spoke he became increasingly agitated. Because he had surprised the staff with this unusual behavior, it was tolerated until it became clear that he was not going to calm down readily. When told that the physician of his choice was being contacted, he agreed to wait quietly in the examining room.

Several of the staff members were then called together to discuss the possible reasons for this change in behavior. Jerry did not appear intoxicated or high. It was known that he had recently been evicted from his apartment for nonpayment of rent and that he had been asked to leave another community agency when he demanded money for rental assistance. Although his aggressive behavior caused concern, it was also the first time Jerry was seen by the staff to have normal feelings of anger. In addition to the staff on hand, a psychotherapist was asked to assist Jerry to examine his behavior. In this setting, for the first time, he requested help. He needed to find a place to live. Even though it was revealed that his recent eviction was known, he fabricated a story about how he had been living with his mother, but that she needed his room for an elderly relative who could no longer afford her current housing arrangement. When questioned about another ten-pound weight loss, Jerry responded that his food money, too, had all gone to his mother.

The social worker assisted in the search. Jerry was also referred to a community home health agency for nursing and social work follow-up. After updating the Social Security benefits, the routine search for subsidized housing was successful. The social worker helped him set up a budget so that his income would cover rent, utilities, and food. Because he had no means of transportation, a plan was devised for a volunteer to bring him to the bank and the grocery store every other week when he received his check. This arrangement worked well for awhile, but soon problems appeared. The volunteer called to say she was concerned because Jerry routinely asked to borrow money from her to supplement the ten dollars per month in food stamps he received. He insisted that his rent and utilities required almost all of his income. Over the past two months, the volunteer had paid several hundred dollars for food and toiletries, and she wondered if there was any way he could get more food stamps or help from other agencies with his rent. While it was gratifying to know that Jerry was receiving an adequate diet, it was not according to the original plan.

At about the same time, his home care nurse reported that he had taken a roommate. He explained that he needed help with the rent. The roomate's reputation in the community centered around his attendance at the early morning methadone programs, and he was believed to buy, sell, and trade drugs.

It was arranged that Jerry's prescriptions be delivered to his home. In addition to enabling a one-pharmacy guarantee, this ensured that Jerry alone would handle the supply. This was successful while Jerry lived alone. Less than a month after the change in living arrangements, Jerry called the pharmacy to say that he had not received his expected delivery. When the pharmacist assured him that the delivery had been made, Jerry claimed that he had not been home, and that the medication must have been left outside of his door and stolen. The signature on the delivery receipt disproved this claim. When he was denied a redelivery, he notified his clinic nurse of the problem. When the nurse did not respond empathetically, he called both the home care nurse and the case manager. Per policy, a new prescription was repeatedly denied.

Jerry calmly explained, "I told the pharmacy that I would not be home at 1:00 to get the delivery. I told them that it was not a good idea to leave it outside my door. I guess they just forgot and left it anyway, and now it is gone. I don't know what I am going to do now. You know that I really need that pain medication."

The nurse's answer was, "Yes, Jerry, we know you have a lot of pain and that it will be hard to not have that prescription. However, the policy is clear. No early refills."

"You have always been there for me," he said. "I think you are the only one who can understand that this was not my fault. I know the delivery was stolen."

"That is not confirmed by the pharmacy, Jerry. The report is that the medication was delivered and that your roommate signed for it."

"What will I do now? I guess I will have to buy some 'on the street.'"

This is a common line used to place responsibility on the health care worker. The nurse calmly answered, "That is your choice and your responsibility. If you are in pain, you can go to the emergency room and the physician on call will give you medication there. In the meantime, you can come into the clinic for a prescription for a nonnarcotic."

When Jerry came into the clinic the following day, it was seen as an opportunity to confront him with some hard facts, emphasizing that the ultimate concern was for his health. He was told, "Perhaps it is time we talked honestly about drugs. How you spend your time, your money, and who you hang with is completely up to you. Please know that all of the people involved in your health care have no responsibility to the police. No one communicates with the authorities about any patients' activities. What we do care about is how these things affect your health and your future. It is our job to monitor your health. To do that we need to know if you are using drugs in order to understand if new symptoms are caused by the prescription medication, the virus, or if it is other drugs you are using. In addition, there are some combinations we will advise you to avoid because of particularly harmful side effects."

Jerry did take the option of going to the emergency room later that evening. In fact, he went to several emergency rooms, obtaining several prescriptions for various narcotics. The outcome was that he was hospitalized for respiratory failure resulting from an overdose. He recovered within a few days and agreed to begin a methadone program and attend Narcotics Anonymous.

Jerry had developed increasingly serious liver problems. He now had intermittent ascites and pedal edema. He would present in clinic with 4+ pitting edema and ask for something to help the swelling. Pain management was a problem since the peripheral neuropathy was worsened by the edema.

When Jerry came to his appointment he was greeted sympathetically: "Hello, Jerry, Your feet are really swollen!"

"Yes," he answered, "I had to walk three miles to get here today because the buses were not running on time and I did not want to be late."

It would have been impossible for Jerry to have walked three blocks with his feet so swollen. He wanted the nurse to feel sorry and somehow indebted to him for his gallant effort to be on time.

The nurse responded in hope of eliciting the real reason Jerry felt he had to spin a yarn. "That is such a long walk. It certainly is a good thing you were able to get here, though."

"You know what I really need is something to make the swelling go down quickly. Do you think you can put in a good word for me?"

Drug users have been self-medicating for as long as they have used drugs. Jerry is a typical example of a recovering drug user. He was not used to any pain, therefore, the pain had to be eliminated by drugs. He was attempting to self-medicate by asking for a drug that he determined was the solution to his swollen feet. If he could engage the assistance of the nurse, his chances of receiving the prescription he wanted would be greatly enhanced.

Because diuretics are so harsh on the renal system and only a temporary solution to a long-term problem, we would first look at other therapies. The first choices would be diet and activity. Jerry's lifestyle was explored by asking, "Have you tried elevating your feet?"

He answered, "Now, by that do you mean above the level of my heart?"

"Yes, Jerry, that is exactly the way to do it. Now tell me about your diet."

He sheepishly looked around the room and said, "I think you must mean the salt thing. Well, I only eat salty things when there is nothing else in the house."

When we heard that there was an opening in the local group home for persons living with AIDS (PLWA), it was presented as an opportunity for Jerry to stabilize his life. He was told that living in this home would involve cooperating with other residents, participating in group activities and duties, and that the clinical staff would administer his medication. He agreed that this was what would be best for him at this time.

While he did arrive the following day with his satchel of belongings, he remained a brief forty-eight hours before he said he had to go out to meet a friend. When present, he obediently followed all the house rules. However, he was absent much more than he was "home." He developed a pattern of returning on a Monday or Tuesday morning, barely able to drag himself into his room. He frequently complained of severe constipation and abdominal distention as side effects of his bingeing. As his face became more drawn in appearance, his weight was falsely increased by fluid retention.

By the time Jerry became homebound, it was feared that he would rapidly succumb to either liver failure or a latent opportunistic infection. Surprisingly, once again he stabilized, and he settled into the group home. A hospital bed and walker allowed him to sleep comfortably and travel independently to the kitchen and bathrooms.

At this point his pain management regime was M S Contin (controlled-released morphine) 300 mg (three 100-mg tabs) twice a day with Percocet (oxycodone), two tabs every four hours for breakthrough pain. The staff dispensed these as prescribed, but often Jerry would say he preferred to adjust his dose, taking only one sometimes and four at other times. He insisted that this was an effective way for him to manage his pain, because some days he felt great and did not need as much medication. "You don't want to overdose me, do you?" he would joke. He received enough M S Contin and Percocet on a weekly basis to match the prescription. By allowing him to adjust his dosage within these limits, it was felt that he would benefit from a sense of control.

After following this regime for over six months, Jerry said one day, "I feel terrible. You promised that I would not be in pain. I needed to take six of the M S Contin this morning and I am still in agony."

Concerned, the nurse asked, "How about the Percocet? Have you taken any today?"

"I don't know. I guess not."

"This is an ongoing concern, Jerry, because, as we have explained, M S Contin works best if taken regularly. The Percocet is the short-acting drug that should be varied as you need or do not need it."

Jerry's facial expression and body language reflected his discomfort. He had been in bed all day. The bedclothes were thrown off of his lower legs, indicating that the weight of the blanket was irritating. He did not often complain.

He said irritably, "I need more M S Contin, that's all."

When the nurse checked, he had no more Percocet available. His delivery was not until the following day. This was unusual, prompting some research into the records. At team discussion, it was thought that the fact that Jerry's dose had not changed in six months was also unusual. Staff then said that he often would ask to have either the Percocet or the M S Contin left on the table for him to take "in just a minute." There did not seem to be a pattern of a need for increased medication following increased activity, as is usually seen. It came to light that, after an afternoon outing with friends, he often needed less breakthrough medication. The outcome was the suspicion that Jerry was selling his pain medication. When confronted, he emphatically denied this. Because he was under the care and responsibility of the staff of the group home, he was obligated to abide by their rules, and he began to take the medication, witnessed by a staff member. Not surprisingly, he required very little Percocet. Also, not surprisingly, he soon had fewer visitors.

Jerry's positive attitude carried him through life. His good nature appealed to the compassion of others. He also cared about what other people thought of him. Manipulation was his way of coping with his hardships and problems. While he occasionally and pleasantly managed to fool others, ultimately he was only fooling himself.

LESSON 4: IDENTIFYING AND DEALING
WITH MANIPULATIVE BEHAVIORS

Manipulation is the overt or covert use of others to meet one's own goals. It is the conscious or unconscious attempt to influence others by distorting the issue at hand for a self-serving purpose (Hamilton, Decker, and Rumbart, 1986). The individual's goal may be as simple as getting attention or affection, or as complex as obtaining drugs. Underlying personality or mental health disorders must be considered during the assessment of unusual behavior. These disorders range from anxiety to a personality disorder.

A form of manipulation is the continual request for services, benefits, and entitlements that disability and dependence can encourage. Through charm or self-pity, the individual plays on the emotions of others. If the patient is allowed to overuse or abuse these entitlements, the patient suffers increased loss of independence and the team suffers loss of credibility.

Undermining the home health team by "splitting" is another form of manipulation. Through the principle of "divide and conquer," the patient can create conflict within the team whereby team members are categorized as being either "good" or "bad." By abruptly and unpredictably favoring different team members, the patient plays people against each other and develops the opportunity to gain the attention, benefits, or medications desired.

Another common manipulative behavior is to request the same service from many sources, resulting in duplication of services. By appointing one team member to address specific types of services, the patient is forced to channel requests appropriately.

Because the lifestyle of illicit drug users involves constant juggling of legitimate and illegal activity, intravenous drug users become experts at manipulating for survival (Baum, 1985). Responsibilities such as a job or school require accountability for frequent tardiness, absences, poor health, and heavy expenses. It is important to expect this behavior, yet not accept excuses when they compromise the plan of care. Harm reduction places the responsibility on the patient. If not, the relationship becomes enabling. If manipulation is not clearly addressed, the behavior will continue and inadvertently be supported.

Ideally, the patient will admit to the true reason for failure to keep an appointment or to follow up on a plan of action. Certain phrases should raise suspicion for the health care worker. They include:

- "You are the only one who understands me."
- "For some reason, I can really talk to you."
- "I have never told this to anyone before."
- "I have complete confidence in you."
- "When the last worker was here, things never were right."

Effective interventions are based on effective communication. Remind the patient that a health care worker has no obligation to report past activities to the police, and that, in fact, prosecution is not an objective. Explain that accurate information about drug use is needed to determine the best medical treatment (Hepworth, 1993). Point out that even convincing lies serve only to waste time that could otherwise be spent looking for solutions to problems. Deal with excuses by clearly stating the boundaries of the relationship. If the patient feels that a health care worker has violated his or hers rights, encourage him or her to register a formal complaint. If this is manipulative behavior, state firmly that you cannot listen to stories about another health care worker.

Other effective strategies are:

- being clear that honesty is necessary in order to provide help,
- giving assurance of confidentiality,
- being nonjudgmental,
- carefully explaining your role as health care provider, and
- focusing on the specific role of your own discipline.

It is necessary to address the problem clearly with the individual, unite team members, and promote each team member's professional role. Consider that what may be actually happening is that the patient is transferring feelings about other relationships to the safe setting of the home health care relationship. If this is the case, the social worker may need to explore the patient's interpersonal relationships and support network. If it is determined that manipulative behaviors are not responding to this united approach, a referral for psychological assessment may be appropriate. Personality disorders are characterized by outbursts of aggressiveness, disregard for the rights and feelings of others, rapid mood swings, excessive attention seeking, impulsiveness, or exaggerated arrogance (Kirkham, 1980). A psychological evaluation may reveal the need for psychological or psychiatric intervention.

Chapter 5

Fasten Your Seat Belt; It's Going to Be a Rough Ride

Mark was sentenced to a two-year prison term following arrest and conviction for possession of heroin. It was during these years that he met the infectious disease doctor who would later see him in the outpatient immunology clinic. On release from prison he followed through with the clinic appointment. His self-confident, friendly attitude was reflected in the way he swaggered into the examination room and said to the physician, "Hey, John! How ya doin' man?" At 6'6" and 240 pounds his physical presence alone was intimidating. He would soon become well known to the clinic staff as a master of manipulation. He would also use intimidation to accomplish his objectives and to try to direct the outcome of a clinic visit. Mark was diagnosed HIV positive six years prior to his first clinic visit. His CD4+ count remained above 500. He appeared to be a healthy, thirty-two-year-old black man.

Because he had not been seen in this clinic before, the nurse conducted a complete psychosocial assessment. The issues and questions centered around drug use, living arrangements, safety, current support, significant others, and future plans and goals.

Mark had not used any drugs in the previous eight months. He had been clean during his years in prison but had relapsed on return to the community a year and a half before his clinic visit. His past drug use was almost exclusively heroin. Occasionally, he injected a combination of heroin and cocaine known as a speedball. He had a twelve-year history of intermittent IV drug use. He agreed that he was likely to relapse again in the future. To help him avoid relapse, people or situations that might lead him to "pick up" (use drugs after a period of recovery) were discussed. People know their personal triggers that lead them into relapse. Discussing them can greatly assist both the patient and the health care team in developing a plan of care.

Mark identified the people with whom he was currently living as triggers. He felt that he was likely to pick up if he stayed in that apartment. He wanted to find a safer place to live. One of Mark's immediate goals was to get his own apartment in another section of the city. The most formidable obstacle was the fact that Mark had no income and no skills. He agreed to cooperate with a community case manager specializing in the area of PLW HIV/AIDS. If he qualified, rent could determined on a sliding scale according to income. Because he had not found a job, Mark could qualify for full rent subsidy. He good-naturedly accepted the offer to be put on the waiting list for a studio apartment.

Planning for the future, Mark was told, needed to include finding employment. He was referred to another case management agency for guidance. Because of his energy and vigor, he would be able to earn a paycheck doing manual labor while considering other options and training programs.

Mark also revealed that he was at risk for endangering his own health as well as the health of others because he had no intention of using condoms. He described sex with a condom as being like "doing it in a raincoat." He felt condoms would be an insult to his manhood. The nurse saw Mark's eyes widen when she said that unprotected sex could expose him to other forms of HIV as well as a variety of sexually transmitted diseases. He listened carefully as she explained the best way to store, handle, and apply condoms. Noting that she still had his attention, she continued by stressing the importance of using only a latex condom and to use a water-based lubricant, since petroleum jelly or oil could weaken the condom, causing breakage. When she offered to demonstrate how to correctly apply a condom on a model, Mark declined, saying, "No way do I need that. I know exactly what I'm doin'!"

Although he was not currently using injected drugs, he admitted that in the past he had shared needles. He said he had never tried to clean his "works." He was surprised to learn that rinsing a syringe, needle, bottle cap, or any other part of the injection equipment with bleach could completely eliminate the virus. The nurse took advantage of his fascination and reviewed the recommended procedure of rinsing all equipment three times with bleach and water and using alcohol to prepare the skin.

As the assessment and the clinic visit concluded, Mark's charming smile was replaced by an aloof attitude as he left the examination room. He was given an appointment to return in one week. During this transition time, it was felt that Mark was vulnerable to relapse and subsequent health care failure.

Since he had grown up in another state, Mark had no family or significant others nearby. He had left his family's home at age fourteen to live with friends. He soon found himself on to the streets, homeless. He had become a loner by choice. He had come to rely on himself alone. He had survived by becoming tougher and stronger than many other guys on the streets. He admitted that he had often relied on his strength to get what he needed.

Working out was part of Mark's daily routine. He had not been idle during his years in prison. Lifting weights and running in the yard gave him a focus. He was proud of the fact that he had survived in prison. He had forced himself to eat the institutional food and avoid the daily irritations and quarrels among inmates. While Mark acknowledged that his history did include violent crimes, he was adamant about his belief that it was better to settle a problem peacefully than by fighting. He was not one to look for trouble.

In order to maintain close contact during this transition period, Mark was given an appointment to return in one week. He returned as scheduled with forms for SSI (Social Security Insurance). All that was required was a doctor's signature. Mark was informed that his chances of eligibility were minimal. HIV disease does not constitute a disability according to state or federal guidelines. Mark responded affably that he needed the form filled out in a manner that would make him eligible. He was told kindly but clearly that the questions would be answered truthfully. When Mark realized that he would not be getting the necessary documentation for SSI, he left the clinic very angry.

Two days later, a paralegal assistant called from a local, free legal aid association wanting to know why Mark's request for completion of the disability forms was denied. He indignantly went on to say that the clinic was legally bound to complete such forms. His tone indicated not only his own irritation, but also seemed to reflect some of Mark's own phrasing. After putting the caller briefly on hold, the nurse was able to collect herself and consider the situation. Knowing Mark's power of persuasion and potentially intimidating manner, she then asked if Mark was present in the legal clinic. The answer was yes. Feeling sympathetic toward this unsuspecting caller, the nurse then asked to speak to Mark. He was indeed still angry and vented his anger over the telephone at the nurse, the doctor, the clinic, and the world, swearing he would sue them all. Only a week later the nurse received a call from the prison asking for Mark's medical records. Mark was incarcerated on parole violation having been arrested for possession of a syringe.

A year later he was released from prison and came directly to the clinic for advice on how to manage his HIV. He was interested in new treatments and smiled charmingly at each receptionist and nurse he passed. He was greeted with warmth, care, and concern. He acted as if he had known he would be welcomed.

An assessment similar to the previous one was done. Similar referrals were made. Mark expressed a desire to stay clean and look for employment. Although he came to the clinic regularly for the next few months, he never had either a job or health insurance. After that, however, Mark again seemed to disappear.

In the immunology center, which specializes in HIV/AIDS, it is not uncommon for Friday afternoons to be an extremely busy time for crisis management. Mark's late afternoon telephone call was no exception. He did not initially give his name. His rapid speech and disorganized thought pattern indicated that his anxiety level was high. Despite this, the nurse soon recognized his voice and wondered whether he wanted to be recognized. Mark, still anonymously, said that he had gone to two emergency rooms as well as a physician and was diagnosed with bronchitis and asthma. When asked about the medications he had been given, he said he had completed eight days of antibiotics and was using an inhaler. His concern was that he was still very short of breath, even when lying down. He said he had not been able to sleep in a week. Finally, he shared that he was also just diagnosed with AIDS. He was asked to come in immediately to be seen by a physician.

Mark responded, "I'm going to die!"

The nurse assured him by saying, "These are symptoms of a kind of respiratory infection. This kind of infection can be treated. It is important that it be treated soon to avoid becoming serious."

Mark anxiously asked, "What do you mean by serious? What could be more serious than dying?"

"There is a kind of pneumonia called *pneumocystis carinii* pneumonia. Many people refer to it as PCP. People with HIV/AIDS are susceptible to this. If that is the problem, there is a treatment for it. The best thing to do now is come and be examined."

"Why didn't the doctor in the emergency room know about this? They took lots of X rays!"

"This type of pneumonia does not always show up on X ray. Sometimes, another type of test will give a definite diagnosis. In any case, it would be best if you could come in to be seen by the doctor."

"Who is the doctor? I know all the doctors there and I only want someone who knows me."

The nurse gave the name of the doctor in the clinic that day, and asked his name. Mark hesitantly revealed his identity. Respecting his wish for confidentiality, the nurse simply acknowledged that she remembered him and assured him that his old records would be available.

When Mark was in the examination room, he had difficulty staying in one place for more than a few minutes. He flitted from sitting in the chair to leaning on the desk, and alternately lying and sitting on the examination table, keeping up a running conversation. Because he was so severely short of breath, his conversation was spurts of pants and wheezes. He was diagnosed with PCP and sent home on oral Bactrim (TMP/SMX) four times a day for three weeks. He slowly improved with each of the weekly follow-up visits.

Unfortunately, what did not improve was his anxiety. Mark had lost approximately forty pounds. Although far from thin, he looked undernourished. He related the onset of anxiety to his diagnosis of AIDS. Intense anxiety is a natural response to such news. Fear, anger, guilt, impulsive behavior, and suicide ideation are other reactions to this critical change in diagnosis. Mark said he had avoided IV drug use but had been using amphetamines recently. He requested the drugs Xanax (alprazolam) and Percocet (oxycodone).

Both medications are easily abused and have a high resale value on the streets. It was explained that because the clinic's specialty was HIV/AIDS, a psychiatrist or psychologist would have to be called to treat anxiety. He was given the names of several doctors who could see him soon. Each week, Mark returned with the same request for the same medication. Each week the explanation regarding the need to use a specialist was given. At that time, he did not follow through with the referral.

It is interesting to note that there are common ways in which patients react to boundaries. Some feel they are a challenge to be broken through or worn down with persistence, by repeatedly requesting the same medication week after week.

Others will try to make the health care worker responsible for their wellness. A typical retort to a refusal for a prescription is, "I guess I will have to buy it on the street." An appropriate answer is, "You do what you have to do. You are responsible for your own choices." Another approach is to say to the health care professional, "I should never have trusted you. I told you I used in the past and now you are holding it against me." After first reflecting to make sure that this is not true, the health care worker should repeat the real reasons for not granting the request. Eventually, Mark did go to a psychiatrist, but would not sign a release of information for the clinic. This impedes continuity of care, but is within the patient's rights.

Mark's next request was for a referral to another doctor in another part of the city. He explained that he was moving and that he would have to take three buses to get to the clinic. Although none were AIDS specialists, he was given the names of several doctors in that area and was told that they could call for his records.

On Christmas Eve, a few months later, Mark appeared in the clinic, anxious and high. He paced around the examination room and rapidly spoke about how sick he had been over the past few days and his conviction that he was going to die.

The physician calmly assured him that he was not dying, while trying to convince him to be still long enough for an accurate examination. As she reached to pick up his wrist, he hugged his arms close to his body. Intending to discover what he might be at risk for, such as a needle site infection, the physician asked, "Have you been using needles?" Mark exhibited some common symptoms of opioid intoxication:

- initial euphoria followed by apathy,
- initial burst of energy followed by psychomotor retardation,
- excessive nodding, and
- pupillary constriction.

Mark startled everyone by jumping off the table as he shouted, "I do not use drugs! And I am insulted that you think I do!"

Concerned, the nurse said, "Mark, it is not like you to act like this. What's going on with you?"

After a short discussion, Mark shared that he had gotten into a fight with some friends and that his girlfriend had left him. Mark's legs were also cut and bruised. He felt depressed and dejected, and he was high on drugs. He did not calm down for long. When he was still refused prescriptions for Xanax and Percocet, he stormed out.

Over the next few weeks, the health care team's concern for Mark's welfare caused them to compile information from several doctors and pharmacies. He was receiving medication from various doctors for anxiety and pain. He had been referred to a community hospice program for home care services. He had convinced them that he was dying, justifying his need for narcotics and tranquilizers. He was being treated as all terminal patients are treated, with medications for comfort. As his use of these medications escalated, however, the home care agency found his behavior increasingly uncooperative. He was found to be high on every visit and unable to communicate effectively. The home care team was concerned for his safety and the safety of their workers.

The turning point for Mark was the day that he struck a tree and wrecked his car. Despite the fact that he walked away unharmed, he realized that he was more likely to kill himself than to die from AIDS.

A contract was developed and signed by Mark and the hospice home care supervisor. It was based on identification of the problems, necessary actions, and a statement of agreement. The goal was to prevent Mark's drug use from endangering himself or others.

The problems identified were:

- being unavailable for home visits,
- not keeping appointments,
- obtaining overlapping prescriptions from multiple doctors, and
- behaving in a verbally and physically threatening manner.

The necessary actions were:

- weekly visits by the nurse and monthly visits by the social worker (either could be more frequent as needed) and clinic visits a minimum of once a month;
- being on time for each visit or calling to cancel the visit within one hour of the scheduled time;
- changing from short-acting pain medication to more efficient long-acting narcotics with adjunctives as appropriate (such as NSAIDs or tricyclics);
- coordination of prescriptions through one physician and one pharmacy;
- signing a release of information to allow the clinic, the psychiatrist, and the home care team to communicate and assess his needs; and
- urine toxicology samples on a random basis.

The agreement read:

- I agree to follow the terms of this contract.
- I am aware that if I do not follow this contract, the home care agency worker will no longer make home visits, and the physician has the right to stop prescriptions.

Over the next few months, Mark was able to secure and maintain a safe place to live. He and the agency have abided by the contract. These clearly stated boundaries enable all the health care workers involved to address his medical and psychosocial needs. His life and story are ongoing. His triumphs are also the triumphs of all the health care professionals who have had the honor of sharing a person's life and life goals.

LESSON 5: RELAPSE PREVENTION

Addiction causes unpredictable and self-destructive behavior. It may be difficult for the compassionate practitioner to observe the patient repeatedly make poor choices. However, it is by anticipating this behavior and by being consistently and readily available that the practitioner can, indeed, help.

Addiction is a chronic and life-threatening disease based on physiological and psychological dependence rather than on a character disorder. Although it is true that an individual makes a conscious decision to use a drug each and every time, the act is compulsive. By definition an addict has lost the ability to control drug use and has become physically dependent on drugs. With opioid addiction, dosages must continually increase due to development of tolerance and decreased intensity and duration of effect.

Expectations of abstinence are unrealistic. Suggesting abstinence implies that the patient has control over the decision to use or refuse drugs. It also implies that the health care practitioner expects the patient to exercise this control. Because both assumptions are wrong, this is a setup for failure. The health care practitioner is expecting more than the patient is able to give. By not living up to these expectations, the patient will suffer feelings of guilt, fear of rejection, and shame in addition to the problems that already exist. As the plan of care fails, the health care practitioner will also suffer from guilt and fear of loss of peer respect.

Further, abstinence may not improve the quality of life. Detoxification causes stress, emotional and physical pain, and abrupt upheavals in lifestyle. Until an individual is strongly motivated, he or she will not begin the process of seeking the support needed to stop using drugs. Until a substance user is willing to accept treatment, the health care practitioner has little choice but to patiently continue to work toward the established goals. Judgmental confrontation may result in the individual leaving the health care system entirely. Relapse is to be expected. Successful detoxification is probably not going to happen on the first few attempts. The individual needs education and support to gain self-confidence and remain motivated.

For the chemically dependent individual, the standard method of dealing with stress is drug use. Stress of any type causes drug craving. The physicians and nurses are a reminder of HIV/AIDS status and, therefore, a major source of stress. Every appointment, telephone call, home visit, test, and contact is a reminder of the illness. By decreasing adherence to a medication schedule and increasing the risk for bacterial infections, drug use further weakens the immune system, stimulating disease progression. The knowledge of this process leads to stress and may further increase drug use.

Projecting what a nonuser might do in a similarly stressful situation or set of circumstances is nonproductive. Because the IV drug user's behavior is controlled by the addiction, it is simplistic to believe that it is possible to simply refuse. Further, this attitude is harmful for the patient and the health care worker because it minimizes the problem.

Objective, nonjudgmental assessment is needed to set up realistic goals. To enable the IV drug user to confront his or her own behavior and chemical dependency, sympathy and moral judgments must be put aside. The individual must gain the confidence to try different coping mechanisms. The relapse prevention care plan must include encouraging confidence through consistent caring and enabling self-help through referral to support groups, counseling, and methadone programs.

The harm reduction philosophy is based on decreasing the amount of risk drug-using behavior may cause. The goals are to protect the health of the addicted individual, the caregivers, and the community. The health care worker can use the established relationship with the patient as a basis for negotiation around controlling harmful behaviors. He or she must:

- Meet the individual at his or her level.
- Learn that individual's level of understanding.
- Establish trust through provision of care and services.
- Be consistent with recommendations.
- Expect or accept active drug use as a part of that individual's lifestyle.
- Assess and recommend treatment for social isolation and depression.

- Teach harm reduction techniques concerning cleaning drug paraphernalia.
- Monitor for side effects and compliance of the IDU.
- Teach nutrition principles; refer to community classes or programs.
- Make crisis intervention available.
- Refer the patient to detoxification and methadone programs whenever ready.
- Refer the patient to recreational activities and support groups.

By incorporating this model into the assessment process, the health care worker has increased chances of success. It is important for the health care worker to remember that individuals have choices. By rising above the desire to control the patient's behavior and drug use, ownership of the problem is given back to the patient. Anticipating the feelings of disappointment or inadequacy when relapse occurs protects the health care worker from emotional burnout.

PART II:
MANAGEMENT FROM
THE HOME HEATH CARE AGENCY

Chapter 6

Back to the Drawing Board

Maureen's life was not turning out the way she planned. Although she had grown up in the poorest of neighborhoods, she always had the basic comforts. She never intended to wake up cold and hungry in a strange room. She never intended to have cravings that drove her wild. She certainly never intended to get "the virus." She knew now, though, that she was closer to the edge than she had ever been before. She admitted she agreed to nurse case management unwillingly, forced by the state. She was thirty-five years old and had been HIV positive for five years.

Maureen had been tested and diagnosed positive for HIV through an anonymous testing site. She had been feeling very tired and was having frequent headaches. She did not feel connected to any one physician or clinic. When she occasionally had a health problem, she went to the nearest walk-in treatment center or emergency room. Most recently, she had been treated for a vaginal infection. She had unsuccessfully tried the usual over-the-counter remedies before she sought medical advice. When she was warned that the infection could become chronic and debilitating if not treated aggressively, she reluctantly agreed to hospital admission for three days of intravenous antiobiotics. Previous to this episode, Maureen's health had been stable other than the cough and bronchitis she tolerated each winter, occasional oral candidiasis, and dermatitis. Knowing she would not consistently take any medication, she had always refused any prescriptions other than a few days worth of pills or an ointment for a specific problem.

At the last hospitalization she was told that her CD4+ count was under 200 and that she needed to begin antiretroviral therapy on a regular basis as well as prophylaxis for PCP if she wanted to live to see age forty.

At the time she came onto the program, Maureen had just given birth to her fifth child; he was HIV exposed. Up to this point, the Department of Children, Youth, and Families (DCYF) had not been involved with the care of the children. However, because this last child was born drug exposed, DCYF was alerted and Maureen lost custody of all her children.

She had a history of IV drug use dating back to when she was a teenager. She also had a history of prostitution. Her other four children had been able to live with her, despite the fact that she had been in and out of prison, because Maureen's mother had been available to care for them on an informal basis. They were now temporarily placed in her mother's custody.

The home care program was faced with the case of a woman who had been in and out of jail, with a history of prostitution and drug use. DCYF had basically told her, "You can no longer have your children. You have done a terrible job of parenting." She was assigned to Sue, a nurse case manager who happened to be new to the agency. Maureen was a true challenge for any case manager, but Sue felt she was up to it. They sat down together and Sue said, "Look, you're going to lose all your kids. There is no doubt about it. If you continue to do the kinds of things that you are doing, you are going to lose custody of all your kids."

Sue spent several sessions in serious conversation with Maureen about what she had been doing and the consequences she was facing. Sue explained to Maureen that if she ever wanted her children to be able to live with her, it was now or never. Sue had an unthreatening way of presenting these painful truths. She said, "This is the way events are going to go if nothing changes. Your mom is going to have custody of your kids. DCYF is going to be very clear about limiting the contact you have with them." She gently but firmly elaborated that the life Maureen's children had led and the situations that they had been in over the past years were unacceptable. She said, "Because of these risks and dangers, DCYF cannot allow this to continue. The oldest kid cannot be left in charge of the younger ones." By their third session within two days, Sue felt there was hope for this family. She said, "We will try to keep you and your family together. In order to do this we need to see some real change happening. Otherwise, this is how it is going to be, this is where those kids are going to be, and this is the role that you are going to play in their lives."

Because this information was presented in a straightforward manner, without criticism or anger, Maureen was able to listen and absorb the information. Maureen needed to hear this from a caring person. She was able to accept the facts and look at her current situation objectively. She was frightened. She was intimidated by DCYF. She understood that DCYF would have no choice but to do their job of protecting her children from an unsafe situation. She understood that she could permanently lose custody of them and, perhaps, no longer see them.

In hindsight, Maureen said, "I came to realize for the first time that I really had HIV and that this might be something that would take my life sooner rather than later. I didn't have time to make any more mistakes. No more second chances." She felt the need to change within herself. "I am going to leave my kids with really bad memories of never being there, of being out on the street and being a drug user." She began to think, "I can straighten my life out now. I want to leave my kids with as many good memories as possible."

Maureen grew up as the only child of a single mother. She and her mother were very close, spending all their spare time together. They would dream about things they would do together when Maureen grew up. They shared meals, holidays, and secrets. That was before Maureen turned fifteen, before she became part of the crowd that experimented with drugs.

As an adult, Maureen's only support was her mother. Her mother had always been there for her and had taken care of the children whenever Maureen was in trouble or away from home. But for the past few years, they had grown far apart. Her mother was very judgmental about the behaviors that had led to her problems. Now, more than ever before, Maureen needed her mother's support. She had had her first child at age eighteen. She now had five children. None of the fathers were involved with her or the children. She did not know who the father of the youngest boy was. She had no parenting skills. But she now said, "I am willing to do whatever it takes to change."

The first thing Maureen did was to go into a five-day detoxification program. When she came out she followed through with the planned outpatient counseling. She also went daily to either an Alcoholics Anonymous (AA) or a Narcotics Anonymous (NA) meeting. Maureen also developed a positive relationship with her outpatient drug counselor. Her counselor became a strong advocate for her in the negotiations with DCYF. She would say to Maureen, "This is what you need to do today, and I will be there for you." Because they were all working together, Maureen felt that she had a support system. She believed that DCYF was also working with her and that they, too, wanted her to succeed in regaining custody of her children.

With the help of her nurse case manager, her outpatient drug counselor, and the AA and NA support groups, Maureen took a leading role in the effort to change her behavior. Because she demonstrated that she wanted to be involved in her children's care and their lives, Sue arranged for her to attend a parenting class to gain formal instruction in how to manage children. She needed to learn basic parenting skills in order to develop a routine that would meet their needs. DCYF was very helpful in coordinating the parent aide and many of the other community resources. The youngest child had recently gone to live in the nursery for children with HIV/AIDS. The staff there was helpful in working with and teaching Maureen how to parent her infant son. They continue today to follow and teach her as he, too, grows up with HIV.

The parent aide is similar to a baby-sitter in reverse. This person came into Maureen's house to demonstrate basic skills such as how to feed, clothe, and manage children. She showed her how to keep the house clean and gave very specific instructions about what goes into a normal household routine. Together they made up a calendar listing the chores and duties that were to be done each day of the week.

Maureen had known only one occupation in her whole life—prostitution. She had no work skills. To find a way to earn a living, she needed to be connected with a vocational rehabilitation counselor, and this completed her schedule, filling the hours of the day when the children were in school. Remaining busy and occupied was very important for her. The rehabilitation counselor helped her to focus on her interests and talents. Interestingly enough, she decided she wanted to be a social worker.

Her first job was in the health care field. She obtained a nurse's aide certificate and worked in a nursing home. She continued to be very motivated. If you asked her what was the driving force behind her ambition, she would have said, "I am concerned about what kinds of memories I will be leaving my kids. I'm not sure if I will be here a year from now. I want to leave them with good memories today." If she did not have children, she probably would never have changed her behavior.

As more resources were tapped, and more people came to believe in her, Maureen gained confidence in herself. With confidence came self-esteem. Maureen knew that she could count on her drug counselor and her nurse case manager to connect her to whatever resources were needed and available. This was of first importance. She needed to feel confident that she could succeed at being straight, at being a parent, and being a responsible member of society. Often, professionals forget the power of self-image and self-confidence. She needed to know that her efforts would not be in vain.

It is not enough to simply say, "Just do this, this way and it will be okay." Skills alone are not enough. Successful integration from "the streets" to the community requires confidence not only in learned abilities, but in self. Without trust and faith in her own ability to succeed, she would have moved from total dependency on drugs to total dependency on other people. If people don't have faith in themselves, when the support system begins to disappear, everything will collapse. One of the differences with her case was that she wanted to change as much as others wanted it for her.

Maureen has maintained her recovery for the past seven years. She continues to amaze all who work with her because she has become a role model for parenting. All of her children are well behaved, well mannered, caring, empathetic children. Maureen is in college now, working toward a bachelor's degree in social work. She has completely turned her life around.

She is also honest with her children about both her past and her present behavior. They know that she has a history of IV drug use and that she used to prostitute. While being HIV positive is a motivating factor, she prefers not to discuss this with her children. She has passed on the job of explaining to her family the implications of the disease to Sue, her nurse case manager. However, she has retained the responsibility of impressing upon them how important they are to her. She admits she has made mistakes. The children have been in and out of her home and other homes. To this day, if asked, she will be very honest in her answers to them. Maureen and her mother also have a better relationship now. They are on friendly terms and spend a great deal of time together.

Maureen has been HIV positive for fifteen years. Because of her HIV-positive status, she sought help from a community-based case management agency. However, it was the work she did with her advocates and counselors that saved her life. She has not had a relapse in seven years following eleven years of IV drug use. Maureen's motivation was fear of losing her children and leaving them with memories of her life on the streets. Maureen's advantage was that of her own, earlier, and stable caring parent. When relearning adult behaviors and responsibilities, she could rely on the core values she was taught in early childhood and redevelop trust in herself and others.

LESSON 6: DEVELOPMENT AND ASSESSMENT
OF COPING SKILLS

Irresponsible behavior can include ignoring or selling essential resources, missing appointments, spending the rent money on luxuries or drugs, smoking in bed, or neglecting family duties. In cases where children are involved, the issues of neglect and abuse are of continual concern and may have legal implications.

Mental and emotional development in the young adult are directly affected by major life changes or events. The developmental stage at which drug use starts may reflect an individual's ability to manage adult responsibilities and cope with normal stress. Other limitations to maximizing functional abilities are intelligence, mental health, sensory acuity, vocational abilities, and communication skills.

The assessment of an individual's coping skills should give insight into previous patterns of problem solving. Knowing what has succeeded or failed in the past will help the practitioner to guide the individual through the current crisis (King, 1993). While everyone has coping skills and patterns, some individuals need to be taught ways to redevelop them. Some need to be shown why one method of dealing with frustration works while another does not.

Home care services and interventions are client-centered. The plan of care develops according to the client's perception of need. This may hinge on the patient's acceptance and management of responsibility. Although patients may verbalize the desire to be a responsible parent, spouse, sibling, partner, employee, or member of a group or community, they may be unable to follow through.

Accomplishment of goals is a proactive process. The practitioner must:

- encourage open communication,
- learn what is important to each individual,
- accept the word of the patient as truth and plan accordingly,
- anticipate potential problems,
- give positive feedback,
- enable easy access to the health care system,
- promote self-esteem,

- gradually increase patient responsibilities, and
- teach and reinforce health-promoting behaviors.

Obstacles to healthy coping skills development are emotional instability, low self-esteem, the desire to please, depression, inability to tolerate frustration, a self-destructive attitude, guilt, and anxiety. Methods to use to develop new coping skills center around building self-confidence and empowerment through knowledge, and support of self-help efforts. Involvement with community action and support groups and skill development will encourage independence.

In varying degrees, the substance user will feel regret and guilt for past behavior and limitations on his or her future. Many have not met the expectations of their parents, siblings, spouses, children, and friends. Many consider themselves to be failures in the eyes of society. Because substance use is a choice before it is a habit, many blame only themselves for the troubles they have experienced. At the time of connection with a home health care system, these feelings may include their current problem of dying and leaving loved ones.

While developing a plan of care as well as a relationship with the patient, it is useful to remember that everyone has a motivating factor that enables change. When accessed, this motivating factor will encourage positive action. Some people are motivated by positive factors such as completion of an event, achievement of an award, personal honor, religion, health, or simply survival. Others are motivated by the desire to avoid occurrence or reoccurrence of a negative event such as incarceration, eviction, drug addiction, loss of job or financial resources, loss of friends or family, loss of health, or dying.

It is often easier for the health care professional to identify the negative aspects of the patient's history. Whether the history is drug use, crime, violence, poverty, or social or business associations, the important fact is that this individual has survived. It is important to focus on the fact that this patient is seeking help *now*. The goal of the initial contact time needs to be identifying one strength the patient has that can be built on.

Visualize a circle. Harm reduction indicates that the patient is met at whatever point he or she may be on this circle. Opening with a statement such as "Let's start with why you are here right now" expresses concern for immediate needs. It is also the first step in the search for motivating factors. If nothing else is apparent, the fact that this patient has survived demonstrates a strength. The next question, "How did you get to this place in your life/this situation?," invites a sharing of immediate, past events. An expression such as, "Look at all the rotten things that have happened. How have you managed to get through all that?" may stimulate a patient to appreciate personal strengths.

By presenting facts in a nonthreatening manner, with an expression of genuine interest, the message is sent that someone cares. General conversation rather than a drill of questions will allow development of a trusting relationship. Gradually sharing information presents the opportunity to understand the patient's problems.

Because patients usually present with one specific, immediate problem, it is important to address that problem, informing them of options as well as limitations to services. The ultimate goal is to build the patient's trust in the agency or organization, rather than in one individual. Health care practitioners will come and go, but patients need to be able to depend on and believe in the organization and medical system.

Chapter 7

In the Eye of the Beholder

Bob was referred to the home health care agency from his medical clinic. He had been released from prison several months before. Prison hospital records showed that he had a low CD4+ count and a high viral load. Since leaving prison, he had been uncooperative with clinic appointments. Because of his high risk for opportunistic infections and disease progression, the physician's request was to discover why he did not continue to seek medical care on a regular basis.

At 6'1" tall and 195 pounds, Bob appeared to be a capable, handsome, forty-one-year-old black man. His strong, healthy appearance belied the fact that he had advanced AIDS, as his blood work indicated. Bob said that recently he had begun to have burning in his lower legs and feet and that he felt he needed help managing his medication.

This enigma of appearance versus medical report raised the question of what else might have been going on in his life. He had obviously not suffered the typical roller-coaster ride of health failures and rebounds. He said he had never had a regular doctor, and had never taken any medication. In fact the only time he had been sick was a brief hospitalization for pneumonia, which did not require follow-up treatment. When asked, he admitted that the severe immune system damage reflected in his blood work could be a result of street drug use. Because he asked for more information about his current health, I told him that his CD4+ count of four and plasma viral load of 200,000 copies per ml was indeed serious, but could also respond to current medication if he was willing to follow the prescriptions.

The initial introduction lasted about half an hour. Bob readily agreed to regular home visits by a nurse who was an AIDS specialist. While the benefits of regular home assessments as well as the limitations of our home care services were explained, he sat nodding his head, agreeing that this was what he wanted. "That is my goal, too," he said. "This is right where I want to be. I want to take care of myself from now on." He continued to say that he was currently attending a methadone program daily and that he planned to continue. At this point a small child appeared. Bob introduced her as his daughter. "I want to be here when my daughter grows up," he said. He was living with his mother. Several times during the interview, his mother came into the living room and sat in the chair opposite the couch where Bob and I were sitting. She nodded in collaboration when Bob stated his intentions. Although she said very little, and showed a genuine concern for his welfare, it was apparent from her facial expressions that she was unhappy.

Their home was in a neighborhood that reflected the daily struggle of the families who live there because they have no other options. While perfectly safe during the day, a plan for visits after dark would have to be made. The stairway to their third-floor apartment was dark, the only light fixture a bulb dangling from the ceiling. However, their apartment was tidy, the counters and floors clean.

Bob's mother said that she had custody of the youngest granddaughter and that she took care of several other, older grandchildren. They seemed well-attended. Occasionally a young girl appeared from another room only to be quickly grabbed by an older child and taken back, laughing happily. Bob said that although he had made mistakes in the past, resulting in the loss of custody of his daughter, he now wanted to be with his family.

The impression Bob gave during this initial visit was that he had both the desire and the potential for his health to stabilize and improve. He had an active support network. He had resources for food and shelter. He was being offered case management services.

Bob was told that he would benefit greatly from resuming normal health-promoting habits including a good diet, a regular medication regime including prophylaxis for opportunistic infections, and a pain management regime. It was explained that this could easily be coordinated by regular, but not necessarily frequent, follow-up in the clinic. Other services available to him included a nutritionist and counseling for relapse prevention either at the methadone program or through Narcotics Anonymous.

The outcome of this first half hour of upbeat conversation was agreement on needs and a tentative plan for short-term goals. As the necessary paperwork was begun, Bob gave the first indication that his agenda was not what it had seemed to be initially. When asked about his current methadone program, he said that he did go regularly, but did not think it necessary to disclose the name of the program or his counselor. He did not think anyone needed to be involved in this area or in what he and his counselor discussed. While this could have been interpreted as a privacy issue, anything that indicates a person has something to hide is a red flag telling a nurse or social worker to ask, "Why?" With a methadone program, the issues could be nonattendance or positive urine tests. Both are indicators of active drug use. While it is understandable that a stranger from a new home care agency should not be entitled to information that would possibly violate a client's probation, lack of information is a concern. Part of risk management is knowing about past and current drug use. Unwillingness to reveal the fact that positive urines have been found probably also indicates that the individual does not intend to give up illegal drug use. Use could amount to a once-a-month binge or it could be a daily situation.

It was reasonable to be concerned that Bob was unwilling to share even the basic information such as the name of the program. It was at this point that he said his most immediate need was simply pain medication.

Bob's referral came on the heels of a clinic visit during which he was prescribed Elavil (amitryptiline) and a nonsteroidal anti-inflammatory drug (NSAID) for pain and Bactrim (TMP/SMX) as a prophylaxis against PCP. He had been disappointed because he felt this was inadequate. In fact, he had not even had these prescriptions filled. He described his pain as limited to his feet and that it worsened with activity, particularly walking. He had to limit his walking to a short block or two. He had formerly been able to walk for miles. When he walked the short distance from the living room to the kitchen, his gait was hampered by the hesitation distinctly typical of peripheral neuropathy.

The standard for pain management starts with the World Health Organization cancer pain treatment ladder. Each step up should be based on the use of a tool. The steps begin with over-the-counter drugs and/or NSAIDs. The progression is the addition of weak opioids for moderate pain. These include codeine, oxycodone, or hydrocodone. As necessary, strong opioids, such as morphine, fantanyl, or methadone can be pre-prescribed for severe pain. "Adjunctive medications are of two types: those with analgesic effects (e.g., antidepressants, anticonvulsants) and those given to central opioid side effects (e.g, laxatives, antiemetics, stimulants)" (Carr and Addison, 1994, p. 22). The addition of an adjunctive may provide relief without increasing the opioid dose.

It was apparent that the clinic physician had a similar concern regarding the situation. The usual pain management evaluation process was explained. Bob was told that because he had not been to one practitioner consistently in the past it was difficult to instantly evaluate his situation. Further, an effective pain management plan could only be put in place if the prescriptions were followed accurately. This process would be expedited if he would participate.

Since Bob denied depression or insomnia, it was also apparent that the prescription for Elavil was to treat the peripheral neuropathy. It was explained that health care workers witnessed its effectiveness repeatedly, that there were only pleasant side effects, and that he actually had nothing to lose by trying this regimen.

The fact that he had not attempted to fill the prescription for Elavil or the NSAID was of concern. This again was a warning about his intention to follow a plan of treatment or a plan of care. When questioned, Bob said, "I tried this before and it did not work. I did not like this medication." He then began to be more forthcoming and said, "I really want Percocet. I know that works for me, because I have tried it. I'll be honest with you. A friend gave me some to try and it worked very well." When asked about the possibility of a long-acting drug such as controlled-release morphine (M S Contin), he firmly shook his head. He had tried that, too, and it had not been effective. Percocet (oxycodone) is renowned for having a pleasant and euphoric side effect. Morphine is as effective at relieving the pain, but without the euphoria. The initial side effects of morphine may actually be unpleasant: nausea or constipation.

These need to be anticipated and treated for comfort and compliance. Chlorpromazine and a laxative should be prescribed and available for the first dosing with morphine.

Bob was told, "It seems that you have every intention of doing the right thing. One thing documented today is the sort of pain you have, when it happens, what degree of pain is happening throughout your normal day, what makes it worse, and what makes it better. We have a good assessment of that at this point. The question is, do you want relief from pain or are you looking for something more?" Bob did not answer this question. He was then told, "Bob, you may have every intention of following a prescription for Percocet. However, other people have not been quite so up-front. They sell their Percocet. You are not going to get Percocet. That is the standard of care now."

The interview ended with Bob agreeing to go to a clinic. The appointment was made for the following week. This would give him time to fill the current prescriptions and be able to determine their effects. The symptoms he was describing were acute. His family agreed that he often limped around the house, demonstrating that he was in pain. He agreed to cooperate with this medication schedule until then. It was important to agree on short-term goals on this first visit.

In order to establish trust, both the patient and the practitioner must agree on the plan of care. This may involve negotiation. It may involve agreeing to disagree. The first goals should be very short-term (such as attending clinic in five days) and very concise (take one medication as prescribed for five days). As these goals are accomplished, there is room for natural progression as trust develops.

Bob did not fill the prescription for the Elavil and the NSAID. He did keep his clinic appointment, however, and, after he had left the clinic, the nurse called to update the home care agency on the outcome. She said that Bob had informed her that he had not filled the prescriptions and that he had no intention of filling them, because he wanted Percocet. He had walked in with an attitude of "give me Percocet or I'm out of here." When confronted with the fact that he seemed unwilling to work within the system and the rules of the clinic, he became belligerent. When he was denied the prescription, he became angry and demanding. Despite the fact that he had legitimate pain, his negative attitude and behavior were seen as drug-seeking.

Such an attitude and behavior should be anticipated. While threatening, intimidating behavior is not to be tolerated, it should be recognized as part of the culture of the chemically dependent patient. This is the way this individual has survived on the streets and in prison. This is the way to cope with frustration. Intimidation may be this person's only defense in daily life. The clinic followed its standard procedure in refusing the prescription, while remaining nonjudgmental about Bob's behavior. He was advised that he could return at any time to get a prescription for M S Contin. However, it was made clear that the only way he would gain cooperation from the clinic was to follow the rules and guidelines about mutual respect.

Bob was called by the home care nurse the next day to ask about the outcome of the clinic visit. Without any prompting, Bob confirmed the conversation with the clinic practitioner. He was no longer angry. In fact, he regretted losing his temper. However, he continued to insist that Percocet was the only medication that would relieve his pain, and he intended to go to another clinic to try to get it. It was again explained that the marketability of Percocet as well as the fact that other drugs were more effective in treating peripheral neuropathy set the standard for pain management. It was emphasized that he was welcome to return to the clinic for a prescription for M S Contin. Bob's conviction that only one drug was the answer, as well as his intimidating behavior, was interfering with effective pain management. It is important that health care practitioners are consistent and do not tolerate intimidation.

Bob said he wanted to try a different doctor. He was given the telephone numbers of two other clinics in the area. The next day he called to say that he had made an appointment at one of them the following week. The outcome of that visit was similarly frustrating for him. He was offered Vicodin (hydrocodone) and an NSAID.

It was now clear that Bob had an agenda of his own. For home care to continue, there has to be cooperation between the patient and the home care team. This may be the biggest difference between home care and an outpatient clinic setting. Because the home care worker comes to the patient, the plan of care agreed upon must be followed if home contact is to be maintained. Without this cooperation, the plan will fail and the services will need to be terminated. In a clinic setting, patients will attend when they feel they want to do so. They come in when they are able to or need to within the clinic's policies for appointments.

Because he did have legitimate pain, it was hoped that he would continue in the home care program. A weekly home visit is usually acceptable to both the patient and the nurse. The patient is not overwhelmed by frequent reminders of his or her illness, yet symptoms of opportunistic infections, weight loss, or nonadherence to or intolerance of a medication regime can be assessed in a timely manner. Although Bob initially agreed, over the next few months he often refused home care visits. Frequent telephone calls to his home were made in an attempt to maintain contact. While his mother benefited from this support, Bob did not.

It is difficult for a home care agency to justify intensive, multidisciplinary team involvement based on a monthly visit. State and federal regulations require documentation of response to treatment, teaching, and/or disease progression to justify reimbursement for each visit. This documentation is labor-intensive for both the field and office staff. If this monthly visit is the result of multiple unsuccessful attempts, it is apparent that the patient is not ready to participate in these services.

Over the next few months, Bob was regularly seen by team members walking throughout the city. He appeared significantly thinner, unsteady on his feet, and blatantly involved in illegal activities. Bob struggled for several months before his mother called to report that he was back in prison. When he is released, services will be available to him. In the meantime, the clinic, the home health care agency, and the prison hospital communicate regularly in an attempt to bring some continuity to chaos.

LESSON 7: WANT VERSUS NEED: DRUG-SEEKING BEHAVIOR

What the patient wants may not be in either his or her, the family's, or the community's best interest. The goal of treatment and symptom management is most effective when mutually determined rather than to satisfy a patient's demands.

While it is important to understand the patient's underlying request and any related problematic issues, it is not acceptable to tolerate bullying verbal abuse or loud outbursts. To tolerate such behavior is to enable the patient to continue. Anger may be intended to intimidate others to get the desired result. In the case of the patient with the dual diagnosis of AIDS/IV drug use this may be entitlements (such as nutritional supplements, food vouchers, bus passes, or rental assistance), equipment (such as a cane or wheelchair), services (such as meals-on-wheels, homemaker, transportation, or social work or nursing visits), or prescription refills. People may try to control the situation by threatening to "fire" the agency or to file a complaint against an individual worker. The patient may harass a worker by frequent telephone calls or insult the worker's ability to do the job.

Following an emotional confrontation, the patient deserves the opportunity to regain his or her composure. It is then appropriate to ask the patient to slow down (rather than calm down). This phrase implies that the health care worker is willing to listen and validates the person's distress. Expressing an interest in finding a solution reinforces the fact that the health care worker does care. This defuses the need to shout. As long as the patient is then able to resume control of his or her behavior, it is important to listen uncritically, without interrupting. Finally, the concerns raised can be addressed according to agency policy.

Hospice has successfully promoted its image of being able to provide effective pain management. This has attracted the attention of the IDU community through the availability of narcotics. Drug-seeking behavior leads to poor pain management. A standardized pain assessment tool is invaluable to assessing the difference between drug seeking and discomfort while promoting continuity. Further, prescriptions should be easy to monitor and yet promote the patient's independence.

While the World Health Organization guidelines are the standard by which medications should be prescribed, the team should determine the quantity and frequency of prescriptions. The attitude of the health care worker may determine how much the patient cooperates with the sharing of information. Because of the threat of loss of probation or parole, loss of housing, and loss of respect, patients have the right to expect confidentiality about issues of illegal substances that they may currently be using (Ashley et al., 1995). It is important to give information on the specific adverse effects of interactions between these drugs and any new prescriptions being considered.

Effective pain management requires confronting the individual who has legitimate pain with the need to set limits. Patients will self-medicate to anesthetize feelings as well as physical pain. This may create a dilemma for the advocate who realizes that the patient will feel the need to resort to street drugs for pain relief if a prescription is not obtained.

Emotional pain can be as debilitating as physical pain. Because instant gratification and relief from all types of pain have been provided for the intravenous drug users through illegal drugs, instant relief is the expectation.

If misuse of narcotics is suspected, prescriptions can be given on a weekly basis. This will keep the patient in weekly contact with the health care system as well as discourage overdosing or sale of these prescriptions. Long-acting narcotics will provide effective relief without the euphoric effect of short-acting narcotics. Refills can be limited to one pharmacy and by one physician. All decisions should be communicated to team members.

Confronting and dealing with the individual who is both seeking drugs and has legitimate pain management needs involves validating the patient's need while setting limits. Safe and effective care depends on this combination.

During the initial assessment period, the patient may express a "need" for tranquilizers, hypnotics, and sleep medication in addition to pain medication. The "need" for food vouchers, rental assistance, and transportation is often the focus of complaints. The team must develop a consistent response to these issues. Each team member must agree to uphold the plan of response to such requests.

Depending on the community resource policy, food and housing assistance funds are usually limited to a set number of requests per year. Cash is never given to patients.

By working to discover what the patient sees as a problem in his or her life, it is possible to mutually agree on a plan of care and to set realistic goals. Some examples of attainable short-term goals are to:

- call for a medical appointment,
- contact a drug counseling center for information,
- follow a short course of prescribed medication to treat a particular symptom,
- keep a food diary for forty-eight to seventy-two hours to evaluate nutritional status,
- go to a local community center for condoms, or
- attend a community-based recovery support group.

If the active IV drug user continues to express a desire for help and is able to complete a short-term goal, it would be appropriate to suggest that he or she:

- attend parenting classes,
- attend a needle exchange program,
- gradually decrease the frequency of the daily drug dose,
- enroll in a drug treatment program, or
- enroll in a detoxification program.

Occasionally a patient keeps an appointment but exhibits symptoms of intoxication, which can include pupillary constriction, slow respirations, slurred speech, falling asleep during conversation, and hypoactive bowel sounds (Jaffe, 1990). Because of impaired memory and judgment at this time, education would be futile and a physical assessment would be skewed. Confrontation should be direct and unthreatening. State the facts. "You are high right now and I cannot talk to you. I will come back when you are sober/straight so we can talk." Another way of dealing with this situation would be to say, "I know you can take care of yourself and that you needed to do this today. However, we have rules about behavior. I hope you will come back when you are sober/straight because I have information about treatments and medication from which you can benefit."

Although it is important to acknowledge a patient's right to continue IV drug use, the health care worker needs to set limits for the safety of the team. Rules to present to the patient for continuing drug use while receiving services include:

- no alcohol or drugs will be taken in the presence of the health care worker;
- no drug dealing in the presence of the health care worker;
- no intravenous access for IV medication will be used for illegal drugs;
- weapons are to be removed from the home during a visit;
- medication will be restricted to one physician, one pharmacy;
- supplies may be limited to daily, weekly, biweekly, or monthly; amounts at the discretion of the practitioner;
- pill counts may be necessary;
- home visits may be restricted to day time hours if a neighborhood is a risk after dark; and
- a caregiver may be asked to meet a home health care worker outside the door.

Helping patients to develop a support network is a key step in a relapse prevention plan. Knowing that there are people available to call upon for help will start the development of alternative coping skills during stressful times. Ideally, the support network will primarily be composed of family members. Frequently, however, the substance user with HIV/AIDS has become estranged from family and must rely on friends, community agencies, or even health care workers for support (King, 1993; Brennen and Dennis, 1996).

Chapter 8

Russian Roulette

Dean swaggered when he walked. He was HIV positive and wanted the best available treatment. He was thirty-five years old, 5' 8" tall, and 170 pounds. He had short, curly, black hair and mellow brown skin. He described his race as "black," but noted that his mother was from Puerto Rico. He had a habit of frequently looking around the room, glancing over his shoulder. He enjoyed lifting weights and working out. He liked to walk everywhere he went because it kept him fit. On his first visit, when asked, he readily revealed the four-inch blade he carried for protection. He seemed proud and tough. He said he had a temper that sometimes got him into trouble.

The clinic policy is clear about weapons of any sort. This policy was explained to Dean and he was asked to leave for the safety of the health care team and the other patients. He was invited to return without the blade. Whether he thought this unreasonable or not, he did not say, but he did comply. When he returned the following day, we made it a point to see him as promptly as possible in return for his cooperation. Weapons are clearly a danger and are not to be tolerated by any health care worker either in a clinic setting or in the home. It is a routine part of the initial assessment to question everyone about ownership and possession of weapons. Although self-protection may mean survival on the streets, the health care setting needs to be neutral and safe.

The projects have a culture of their own. Dean grew up to respect hard work and to expect tough times as a teenager. He did not have many fond memories of his childhood environment. Growing up meant proving his manhood. By the time Dean was nineteen he had fathered two children and had one gunshot wound in a leg and a stab wound to one shoulder. Although he said he had never had any intention of settling down with any one woman, he said emphatically that he had provided financial support for the basic needs of his children.

To look at Dean you would not think he had a care in the world. His cutoff jeans and T-shirt fit his personality. However, the reality of his story was quite different. His hands were always in motion, repeatedly clenching into fists, a clue to his constant readiness to meet any challenge. He had gone to prison for three years in his late twenties for assault and robbery. When he returned to the neighborhood, he found that both of his children had moved with their mothers to unknown communities. Although he was eventually able to locate them, he had no money to travel or even to telephone. This was a source of frustration for him.

Dean had multiple risks for HIV infection through both intermittent IV drug use and unprotected sex. Whether these continued to be a risk for him while he was in prison, he did not say. What he did say was that he learned to be "strong" and had spent a great deal of time lifting weights while incarcerated.

Soon after being released from prison, Dean fell in love again. This time, he said, he had truly intended to settle down. While they never had an official ceremony, Dean referred to Alicia as his wife. It was not until Alicia was three months pregnant that she began having severe gastrointestinal and respiratory problems that quickly led to her hospitalization and diagnosis of AIDS. Their child lived only a few months after birth, and Alicia died a year later. Dean delayed being tested himself until after Alicia died. He was not surprised to find that he, too, was HIV positive. Dean carried a picture of Alicia and a newspaper clipping with his infant son's picture. Because he had devoted himself to their care, their memories were a source of both grief and pride.

With or without a knife, Dean thrived by living on the cutting edge of daily excitement. After Alicia died, he moved in with his sister and her family. After only a few months he was asked to leave, however, because he and his brother-in-law disagreed about almost every aspect of daily life. Dean moved into a third-floor apartment in an abandoned building. He had a small table and one chair and slept on a pile of blankets. He had already befriended a young woman and they shared the living space. One aspect of their relationship that Dean did not like was her addiction to heroin. He said he was no longer into that and that although he enjoyed her company, he wished she would give up the drugs. He said that his only indulgence was that he "enjoyed a few beers from time to time." As innocent as this may seem, for a person who lives on the streets it can be detrimental. There is no having just one beer, one tranquilizer, or one snort of cocaine. Drinking and drugging invariably lead to venting the anger and frustration that accompany poverty, illness, and real or perceived discrimination against minorities and people living with AIDS.

His story was gradually revealed over the following months. When his CD4+ count dropped from 300 to below 50, he was given monthly prescriptions for Bactrim (TMP/SMX) and AZT (zidovudine). The hope was to keep him coming around for a monthly checkup in the clinic. He often had unexplained bruises. He vaguely spoke about "protecting his turf." During this time, there were opportunities to discuss safe sexual practices, hygiene, and referral to the local HIV/AIDS chapter for free community services.

When Dean came to the clinic without an appointment and before he needed his monthly prescriptions, we knew something was very wrong. He reported having increasingly severe headaches for the past week. He also complained of fever, fatigue, and memory loss. He was sent for an emergency CAT scan and a lumbar puncture. The diagnosis was cryptococcal meningitis, requiring inpatient, intravenous amphoteracin B therapy.

Three weeks later, although he had lost almost forty pounds, he was greatly improved and eligible for discharge if he could continue the IV therapy at home. However, without a telephone or electricity in his third-floor apartment, his living quarters did not meet the minimum standard for home IV therapy. On the other hand, he was not to be talked out of the opportunity to leave the hospital. He went home on oral Diflucan (fluconazole). He was referred to a hospice home health care agency with the expectation that his chances of survival were poor.

He did survive. It was at this point that he began making the daily one-mile jaunt to a local group home for patients with AIDS. His intention was to make contacts and to move in as soon as there was an available apartment. However, although he described his behavior as determined, it was seen as demanding and rude. Unfortunately, he did not treat the staff there with the same respect that we had seen at the clinic. He soon was denied the privilege of visiting and even use of the telephone. His quick temper did not allow him a smooth ride into middle age.

Not only did Dean survive, but he actually thrived after his discharge from the hospital. He decided to leave his girlfriend even though he knew she would be angry, because she depended on his SSI income. He left her one night following an argument, walking out with only the clothes on his back and his prescriptions. He convinced a cousin to take him in until he could find an apartment. Within a month, with the help of the social worker and a written recommendation from the medical staff, he was able to find a rooming house with one bath per floor. He cautioned that no one was to know his new address, especially his former girlfriend. He said that she would pursue him for his money. However, within a few weeks it became evident that there were other reasons for his secrecy. Apparently, Dean had made promises to her that her older brothers intended to see that he either kept or suffered the consequences. Once again, Dean began carrying the blade and coming into the clinic with abrasions and bruises.

Over the next several months, Dean was cooperative and punctual for all his appointments. He was seen weekly for one month and then tapered off to once a month. He was completely free from all symptoms of cryptococcal meningitis. He developed anorectal condylomata, which required painful cauterization on a regular basis. While this temporarily restricted his walking, he soon resumed and increased his distances up to five miles a day.

Dean announced that he intended to get a job. He wanted to earn enough money to travel. Despite his good intentions, his determined style of forcing his wishes got in the way. He found a job cleaning up after hours in a pizza parlor. The benefits were that he could eat all the pizza he wanted and he was paid under the table. However, after only a few weeks he said he resented having to wait until all the customers left to begin his cleanup and that he deserved more money. True or not, he began to express discouragement and claimed that he was being discriminated against because he had AIDS. Bad news travels quickly, and Dean's misfortunes were soon known throughout his small community. Dean applied for several other jobs, and was repeatedly rejected for each one.

During this time, Dean did not remain completely out of trouble. He called to complain to his social worker that the electricity had been turned off in his building and that without the refrigerator, all of his food had spoiled. He wanted to know how he could get the landlord to replace it. He had a long list of frozen meats as well as fresh food items he wanted to claim. Making a home visit, the medical social worker was surprised to find the refrigerator on its side with the door unhinged. Dean explained that he had had a disagreement with a neighbor, but they had resolved the situation. While tipping the refrigerator back up onto its feet, the social worker discreetly asked more about the incident and discovered that the food in the refrigerator had possibly been stolen during this altercation. Further, the loss of electricity had lasted less than four hours. When confronted with the likelihood of eviction if he pursued his questionable claim of spoiled food, Dean changed his mind.

While he denied having resumed a relationship with his former girlfriend, she continued to be a source of trouble for him. During a routine home visit, he was found sitting dazed on the edge of his bed/couch, with a three-inch gash across his forehead. He explained that his former girlfriend had hit him with a lamp when he refused to give her any money. He temporarily dropped his tough-guy attitude as he complained that her brothers would be waiting for him if he went outdoors. However, when questioned about the need for police intervention he straightened up, declaring that he "wasn't afraid of anyone!" Although he had stopped the bleeding with a towel, he agreed to go to the emergency room for sutures.

About a week later he received an eviction notice, after his former girlfriend was found injecting heroin in the common bathroom. It was avoided, however, because he was able to contract with the landlord, through the community social worker, that he would avoid all contact with her in the future and that the drug use would not happen again.

Dean lived from check to check. He did not know how to plan for even the near future. When his rent and utilities were paid, he spent the rest of his monthly income on anything but food, clothes and necessities. If he could borrow a few dollars, he would buy iced coffee or beer. On one home visit he proudly displayed a new gold ring. By the next week, the ring was gone. When he was given a calendar to mark his appointments, he said he did not own a pen or pencil.

Dean struggled with his desire to regain self-respect through financial independence and to maintain his reputation within his community. Despite his own recovery, he repeatedly suffered the consequences of his choice to continue to interact with others who actively used drugs. The violence inherent in this lifestyle put him in harm's way. It will always be an unanswered question whether, had he lived, his energies could have been channeled in a way that would have promoted his own health and safety as well as those around him.

LESSON 8: THE PREVALENCE OF VIOLENCE
AND RISK-TAKING BEHAVIORS

The lifestyle of HIV/intravenous drug users is inherently mixed with violence. Violent behavior is an accepted part of the risk taking the intravenous drug user faces daily. People "infected with HIV are disproportionately affected with violence in their everyday lives" (Seals, 1996, p. 91). The act of intravenous self-injection is, like any physically violent act, invasive and painful. To accomplish such an act requires powerful motivation. The desperation of addiction drives individuals to do whatever it takes to fulfill their needs and desires. Because heroin is illegal, the rules of the game in America are a setup for violent behavior (Wartenberg and Samet, 1992). The purchase, sharing, and environment of intravenous drug use are fraught with violence. The social stigma of HIV/AIDS is accompanied by the threat of violence through anger and rejection (Miller, 1990).

Violence is more prevalent in lower socioeconomic communities. Families who live in poverty often witness violence in the form of assault, robbery, child abuse, spousal abuse, rape, drive-by shootings, and prostitution (Fontanarosa, 1995). Many within this population are victims of childhood trauma and domestic violence (Cull, 1996). Children are primed to accept this behavior, and they enter adulthood through the door of sexual risk taking and social marginalization.

Domestic violence affects more than one million women each year. Women who have been victims of sexual and physical abuse make up a significant percentage of the HIV/IDU population. Interventions should empower women to realize their options within the legal, medical, and social service systems. Due to the risk for escalation of violence, it may be safer for a woman to stay in a violent relationship. Health care workers need to recognize their role as educators. Through support and encouragement, women can develop skills to maximize their potential for education and career opportunities.

"But violence is beyond being pervasive. Violence is seductive, alluring, and perhaps addictive" (Seals, 1996, p. 91). Because the neighborhood bully can control those around him, because there is a sense of security in control, and because being safe in a violent world means having superior strength, control requires violence. The superior individual thus can gain control of his or her circumstances and the respect of peers. In a society that rewards the powerful, condemns the weak, and offers little hope to those in the middle, it is not difficult to understand the motivation for this struggle.

Our urban communities, "disproportionately affected by the HIV epidemic" (Singer, 1994, p. 932), are populated by families living in poverty. Through inferior education, poor access to individualized health care, and social marginalization, the urban poor are ill equipped to manage the ever-increasing stresses of life today. A common reaction of an IDU to a diagnosis of HIV is to escape through escalated use.

In addition to the high risk for HIV exposure and transmission, these people are also unprepared to manage their anger toward society for their plight. Anger has long been identified as a normal or natural part of the process of grieving. It is therefore no surprise that anger is a common reaction to both the diagnosis of HIV and to the individual with the disease (Phillips, 1996).

Violent thoughts and behaviors are to be expected but not tolerated in the health care setting. One solution is to contract with the individual about behaviors that will not be accepted. The contract should address an individual's usual response to stress or frustration and their ideal, expected, and necessary behavior in the presence of the health care worker. The contract needs to identify specific, witnessed behaviors that have caused concern. Expectations for behaviors that ensure employee safety should be clearly stated. The agreement must include consequences of recurrence of these behaviors. Both parties then sign to indicate their commitment and understanding. The contract must be based on truth rather than rumor. The goal must be to establish a mutual, trusting relationship rather than to simply rid the agency of the patient. Consequences of breaking the contract could include ending the visit immediately, denial of refills on prescriptions, postponement of health care or social services, or termination of services with referral to another provider.

To promote employee safety, all team members need to be immediately informed of a potential dangerous situation. To deter confrontation, interventions can be performed by two employees and/or in the presence of a friend or family member. Individuals who escalate a situation should be asked to leave prior to the arrival of the health care worker. Weapons of any sort are to be removed from the home prior to the visit.

Nurses, social workers, and HIV educators can be role models for activism in community safety. They are in key positions to directly intervene in the vicious circle of violence. Through identification of individuals at risk, community education, and referrals to community-based agencies, health care workers can be the voice of prevention. As advocates for individuals afflicted or affected by HIV/AIDS, home health care workers are a vital link to an elusive and complex medical system.

Chapter 9

Secrets

"My favorite time of year is the summer. I like to lie on a sandy beach on a very hot day. Mostly because I really love the beach. I like to have a cold soda and feel the hot sun on my back and legs. I could lie there for hours enjoying the sounds and smells. Lately, though, the beach has been getting too busy and crowded. It's nice to be around people sometimes, but I like to have some time by myself.

"I had a dream about the beach. In my dream the tide was always going out. The sand was always wet rather than warm and dry. Just a few feet away from me, toward the water's edge, were lots of little holes. And there was constant activity, little squirts, coming from these holes, and from a lot of new holes. I figured out that they were clams, popping up and disturbing the quiet, smooth sand. They wanted to squirt out. At first, I got up off my towel and stepped on the new holes in the sand. But soon there were too many of them. As fast as I could step on one hole, I'd see three or four more popping up right nearby."

Martha was diagnosed as HIV positive nine years before she began regularly attending the clinic. She had been tested anonymously and had not shared her diagnosis with anyone. Martha had been denying her illness for a long time. She said, "It's not a problem. Sometimes I think about telling someone, but not now. No one needs to know yet." Denial enables Martha to forget her illness.

As she speaks, Martha's long reddish-blond hair repeatedly falls across her white face. She unconsciously pushes it back behind an ear and flicks stray strands away from her face. Her casual dress of jeans and loose top make her look younger than thirty-five. She recently gained fifteen pounds, adding to a somewhat unkempt appearance.

Over the past few months, Martha's visits to the clinic have become more frequent. When asked, "How are you?" her response is consistently negative. She suffers from ongoing headaches, earaches, backaches, and upper respiratory infections. While these ailments vary, they never resolve.

Martha's single, obvious disfigurement involves her right hand. The fingers curl together, just short of closing. Her wrist remains flexible and functional. She supports this hand in her lap when sitting. Multiple evaluations have not revealed the cause. Physical therapy has not enabled her to regain use of the hand. This affects her writing and her ability to perform many household tasks.

Because she virtually did not attend school past the third grade, Martha is functionally illiterate. This came to light when she called to ask for a new prescription for Vicodin (hydrocodone). When asked, over the phone, to read the label and the number of pills originally dispensed, she gave inconsistent information. When the pharmacist was called to clarify the prescription, the inconsistencies became confusing. Martha finally admitted that she sometimes had difficulty reading "the small print." Over the past three months, she has been taking courses to learn basic English and mathematical skills. Although her attendance is erratic because of her frequent ailments and dislike of public transportation, she is now better able to manage her medication.

To maintain her secret, she must justify her frequent ailments. Intense back pain was diagnosed as being related to a kidney stone. She was booked for lithotripsy and given a prescription for M S Contin (controlled-release morphine) and Vicodin. Following treatment, she was told that there was one stone left behind, but that it was stable and would not cause her any pain. After several weeks of pain management, the back pain had not resolved. In fact, the same pain had intermittently intensified. Only after repeated X rays verified that this stone was stable did she agree to be weaned off the pain medication.

After repeated complaints of a headache, she was treated in the emergency room with an injection of intramuscular Demerol (meperidine) followed by a week of oral Dilaudid (hydromorphone). When the results of an MRI were normal, Martha's reports of headaches stopped immediately.

Martha frequently complains of weight loss. Typically, when asked about her appetite, she replies, "I just can't eat." One focus of the home health nursing care plan is evaluation of diet and nutritional status. Martha's nurse case manager was concerned when she reported a weight of 115 pounds, knowing that she had been 128 pounds the week before. A call to the clinic revealed that Martha's weight had been maintained at 128 pounds. Two days later, on a follow-up visit, the nurse had the same conversation about appetite and weight. When she reminded Martha of the clinic's report on her visit two days earlier, Martha shrugged, saying, "Oh, I forgot."

Martha is chronically but intermittently afflicted with painful external genital and rectal herpetic lesions. The treatment is oral and topical Zovirax (acyclovir). If Martha interrupts this regime, the lesions flare up within a few weeks.

Martha shows no interest in knowing the current status of her disease. She does not know her CD4+ count or her viral load and shows no interest when tests results are revealed, whether good or bad.

Martha lives with a longtime friend. They met over twenty years ago and have shared housing off and on ever since. They have lived in their current apartment for the last several years. Martha's disability check is their only dependable income, although Nick finds temporary jobs from time to time. It is a mystery how Martha and Nick survive on her disability check. They both freely describe the fine meals Nick prepares. Last Father's Day, Martha gave Nick a handsome watch. They have a new color television. Martha volunteers that the local grocery store "always passes out meats." Apparently they are equally generous with pet food, cleaning supplies, and house plants, which are plentiful in their apartment. Martha also claims that the Salvation Army insists on giving her money. She volunteers in the store for an hour and they insist on paying her for a full day. Their church friends are also generous with money and donations of food or clothing.

In the beginning of their relationship, Nick provided clients for Martha as a prostitute. The money was spent almost entirely on drugs. When asked to describe her life in general during those years, she shrugged innocently and stated, "It was an easy way to get money. We could get all the drugs we wanted." Their drug of choice was freebase heroin.

To take this conversation a step further, she was asked how she thought Nick would react to the knowledge that she was HIV positive. She replied, "Nick just found out that a nephew of his has AIDS. Now he won't have anything to do with him." Nick's educational background is not known, but he has been seen reading the Bible. He drives and maintains his car. He has a wealth of information about home remedies for Martha's multiple ailments. He, too, is street-smart. This raises the question of how Martha's HIV status can be unknown to her intimate partner.

Martha's nurse case manager asked, "What does Nick think is wrong with you?" It was not a secret that Martha had multiple appointments, tests, and a visiting nurse from a hospice agency. Martha answered, "Nick just thinks I have kidney problems and stones. He doesn't know what hospice means. He just thinks I am having a hard time with my health." By withholding her diagnosis from Nick and her family, she can pretend the HIV/AIDS is not a problem, enabling her denial. If Nick were to know, it would become real. On the other hand, the multiple ailments validate her precarious physical health as well as provide the much-needed psychological attention. Martha has been known to call 911 for a toothache.

When Martha was nine years old, her mother died. This tragedy was complicated by the fact that her father, a former police officer, pushed her mother down the stairs causing the death. Both Martha and one older sister witnessed this event. She remembers that her mother had recently announced that she was pregnant with her ninth child.

Martha has a picture of her mother in her living room. They bear a striking resemblance, except that, even now, Martha appears much younger than her mother. She recalls being put into foster care soon after her mother's death. She states she rarely attended school and officially dropped out at age sixteen. During the years in foster care she lost contact with her brothers and sisters. As adults, they do communicate, but irregularly. Her father has since died; he was never prosecuted for his part in the death of his wife. Martha has very few memories of these childhood years, and what she does remember is all bad. She was raped in several of her foster homes. She remembers shame and isolation. At nineteen, Martha had a son. He lives now with her older sister in another state. She hears either about him or from him occasionally, but does not know much about his life.

Nick's ethnic background is African American and American Indian. Indian artifacts decorate the living room walls. He never fails to smile a greeting, displaying a single remaining tooth. Nick's politeness and good nature seem to be shared with the community in general. He has pictures of his nineteen children displayed around the apartment. They range in age from six months to thirty-two years. His oldest daughter is a grandmother herself. He keeps busy both around their apartment and working on his refurbished 1960 Oldsmobile.

Martha's contact with her family is limited because of her relationship with Nick. Her siblings disapprove "because he is black." Nick's family, she says, are equally unhappy and do not like her "because I am white."

Both Nick and Martha are in recovery for alcoholism and IV drug use. They have both been clean for the past year. Martha attributes staying clean to having found God. When she gets a craving, Martha says, she simply reads the Bible and is able to overcome the urge. They attend church services regularly. She is proud that she "made communion" about six months ago. Unfortunately, the fact that she and Nick live together, unmarried, is a problem for her friends in the church.

When she shared this information with her nurse, it was seen as an opportunity to explore their plan for safer sex. Because Martha has never shared her HIV status with Nick, there is concern for his health. On the other hand, never having had a conversation about HIV with Nick, she has no way to know his HIV status. However, for the purpose of education about condoms or other safer sex equipment, it is not necessary to know Nick's HIV status. When asked about using condoms, Martha replied, "Oh, I don't need them. Nick and I never have sex. In fact, I haven't had sex in twelve years. Besides, the church and our religion say that couples who are not married should not have sex." While the apartment does have two bedrooms, a recent home health care team meeting shared that, at least on one occasion, during an early morning visit, Nick was seen in Martha's bed. Martha was gently confronted with the fact that Nick was at risk for HIV infection and that she could be exposed to further infections. She was informed about the anonymous partner notification program through which Nick could be advised of the fact that he was exposed to HIV.

Martha's stories about her past are filled with inconsistencies. She always appears to be forthcoming with information. It is apparent, however, that if she does not remember or care to share some information, she changes the details. During this discussion, Martha insisted that she had no need for condoms. She said she was fully aware of when and how to use them, but she had not worked as a prostitute nor had any sexual relationships for the past twelve years (the period of time she has been HIV positive). On the other hand, it is known that she was incarcerated for prostitution six years ago. Her reluctance to discuss or reveal the actual cause of her multiple health problems raises a concern about her understanding of their origin and potential transmission.

Martha fabricates what she would like to be true. At this chronic, progressive stage of her disease, she is having increased fatigue and increased frequency of sinusitis and upper respiratory infections. With a CD4+ count of under 100, she is diagnosed with AIDS and is closely monitored for symptoms of opportunistic infections. At the same time, her history of drug use and frequent requests for narcotics complicate her plan of treatment.

Martha is committed to hiding her diagnosis from her family and friends. Hiding her medications and medication list requires endlessly checking counters and table tops. She prefers to keep all of her medication tied in a bag on the top shelf of her closet. She refuses to accept any appointment cards or to write any appointments on her calendar.

When it was first revealed that Martha had not shared her secret with anyone, the need for precautions with body fluids was discussed. She was asked, "What would you do if you cut yourself and needed first aid?" Martha glibly described preparing a weak bleach solution to clean up any blood or spills. She adamantly declared that she would not let anybody touch her or be exposed to any cuts. The fact that she is knowledgable about precautionary measures in these situations belies her ruse of naiveté.

One of the services offered by the home health agency is transportation by volunteers to and from medical appointments. While other avenues are available, this service is naturally preferred by patients because of convenience. While it is not possible to offer this service to Martha for daily classes, accommodations are attempted for her medical appointments. With the frequency of her appointments, this is a challenge. When she requests a ride, Martha is questioned about Nick's availability. Her response usually is, "He has to work that day." When a volunteer is unavailable, Nick mysteriously and invariably appears, ready to take her.

Martha's negative attitude seems to be a way of life, resulting in constant complaints about people, places, and events. Her anger overshadows her judgment. She complains frequently about the neighborhood and about the neighbors, although the apartment and neighborhood are seen as acceptable by the home health team.

When the pharmacy once left a routine delivery of medication with her neighbor, she was irate for weeks. When Nick is absent, he becomes the object of her anger.

Usually, the intimate nature of the relationship between a patient and a home case nurse leads to a bonding over time. This has not happened with Martha. When going on vacation, the nurse informed Martha that another nurse would be coming in the following week. Martha replied that she did not care who it was that came. She is not connected emotionally with anyone. She does not say "please" and "thank you." While willing to answer any questions asked about either her health or personal life, Martha does not elaborate nor offer details. She does not initiate confidences.

Martha's wish for a peaceful day on a warm sandy beach is spoiled by the reality of the ebbing tide. Just like the clams squirting up from the sand in her dream, the thousand excuses and fabrications she has used over the last twelve years are becoming harder to control. She has difficulty explaining her increasing health problems. She has lost track of exactly what is true. Multiple tragedies in childhood and adolescence have forced a premature entry into a cruel adult world. It would seem that she lacked the opportunity to fully develop the ability to love and trust. In her favor, she has learned survival skills, developed a new faith, and has chosen to challenge herself with education. With these, the hope is for a new respect for herself and others.

LESSON 9: VOLUNTARY DISCLOSURE:
ETHICS OF CONFIDENTIALITY
WITHIN THE COMMUNITY

Health care workers need information to provide effective care. With this information comes the moral responsibility to respect the patient's decision to reveal or withhold a diagnosis of chemical dependency or HIV-positive status to others. Fear of disclosure to friends or family is rooted in concurrent fear of personal rejection, fear of isolation, fear of loss of financial resources, and fear of violence.

First is the fear of personal rejection. By revealing this secret, a person risks abandonment by significant others. At the very least, it is a frightening thought that your neighbor might refuse to speak to you or that you might find yourself sitting alone in a church pew. It is even more intimidating to consider that a health care worker might refuse to participate in your care. The fear of discrimination in the school system or during social activities is particularly intimidating for HIV-positive women with children.

Refusal to care for patients with HIV/AIDS is both unethical and (as of 1992) illegal. The position of the American Nurses Association is that a nurse can refuse to care for an individual who is HIV positive only if the risks exceed the responsibility of care.

A second fear is that of isolation. If an individual's friends and family react negatively to the disclosure, the patient may find he or she is avoided altogether. The health worker can offer to involve significant others in support groups either individually or with the patient. Being firmly established within a support group prior to revealing a status will be helpful in case a significant other does, indeed, abandon the patient, even temporarily. By fostering self-respect and treating the patient as an equal, a health care worker can be seen as a role model. Often people have developed a self-imposed isolation through guilt and powerlessness. Women, especially, are at risk of feeling that they do not deserve help.

A third fear is loss of financial resources. This is based on fear of losing a job or financial support from a significant other.

Many times the fear of violence is well-founded. Because of social dynamics, there may be little a health care service network can provide other than support in the clinical setting. The offer to be physically present during the disclosure process may provide protection for the patient who faces real, physical violence. Any local abuse hot-line numbers as well as a referral to an appropriate agency for personal safety should be readily available.

The fear of violence may indicate how a patient believes he or she would react or may be based on past reactions of the significant other. Health care professionals must take a patient's fear seriously, develop skills to assess the potential for violence, and establish a climate in a controlled setting for patients and families to discuss their needs.

By continuing to keep his/her HIV-positive status a secret, the IDU may be repeatedly and knowingly exposing a significant other to the virus. The case of *Tarasoff vs. Regents of the University of California* (1976) addressed the "legal and clinical problems in treating life endangering clients." The Tarasoff decision has legal implications for all health care workers treating any patient with a potentially life-endangering diagnosis. For the HIV/AIDS/IDU the life-endangering aspect is transmission of the virus. The outcome of the Tarasoff decision is that the health care worker or therapist must determine that the danger is real and imminent and that there are actual victims. Some patients may claim that they have indiscriminately and purposely infected others (VandeCreek and Knapp, 1989).

Courts have found that negligence hinges on the assessment for the "potential for violence" or harm. Health care practitioners need to be aware of their legal obligations and limitations.

One reason to respect a patient's confidentiality regarding their HIV-positive status is to maintain contact with them. Premature disclosure may result in losing the trust of the patient. Loss of trust and contact would result in a potential danger to other, unidentifiable persons in the community. Several states have partner notification programs that allow trained counselors to respond to a patient's request to inform another person of exposure. This is done without revealing the identity of the patient, avoiding direct contact with a former partner.

The benefits of sharing a problem (or a life-threatening diagnosis) may need to be made clear through education and support. People will practice the value system learned during childhood.

Automatic responses to a diagnosis of HIV/AIDS may be (1) do not show vulnerability, (2) do not admit mistakes, or (3) do not ask for help (Marlin, 1989). The offer of a safe, supervised setting may provide relief from the stress of anticipation of the emotional reaction of a partner, friend, or family member.

Explain that disclosure will result directly in increased communication between the patient and his or her significant other, more effective health screening, and availability of referral sources and resources, decreased emotional stress, and decreased need for medication related to that stress.

The stress of not disclosing one's HIV status, especially to a significant other may be worse than the actual disclosure event, although the longer a patient has maintained the secret, the easier it will have become to cover it up. As time goes on it may be more difficult to disclose both the HIV-positive status and the coverup. Keeping this secret involves hiding appointments and prescriptions. It means neglecting necessary medical follow-up and ignoring symptoms of deteriorating health. It means living with the guilt of having acquired the virus and potentially transmitting it to someone the patient loves. It means obstructing the normal grieving process that goes along with having a terminal disease. In addition to encouraging disclosure, other ways of offering support are to:

- affirm health care practitioner availability,
- encourage a positive attitude toward daily events,
- have a list of community support groups available,
- be knowledgeable about resources and activities,
- offer hope for better health through medical intervention,
- inform of alternatives for stress management,
- anticipate the charge in relationships, and
- offer support for spiritual distress.

Effective counseling can encourage voluntary disclosure. Exploring and evaluating the reasons for not disclosing a diagnosis to a significant other should be the focus of the counseling. Encourage the patient to reveal the reasons for withholding this information. Offer to call the significant other or to accompany the patient and assist with the disclosure.

Anxiety and fear around the fact that HIV/AIDS is a life-threatening illness needs to be anticipated. While it is important to respect an individual's desire to not discuss dying, it is equally important to be prepared when the patient is ready or receptive to this subject. By defusing a patient's fears about treatment, symptom management, or life expectancy, we can ease emotional pain and suffering.

If we are ever to break the stereotype and discourage the stigma of HIV/AIDS, we must support those who have the courage to share their HIV-positive status openly. We must then work to create a nonthreatening environment that allows open discussion of the disease and treatments.

Chapter 10

So, What Now, Babe?

Cindy rolled over to look at the clock next to her bed. It was only 4:30 a.m. Too early to get up for the methadone program. As she settled back into bed, she considered once again how remarkable it was that she awoke at all. Today she was able to smile at the thought. The familiar struggle with depression and negativity was not going to happen today. Some days, however, the same thought brought tears to her eyes and a heaviness across her chest.

Two years before, Cindy was told her CD4+ count had dropped below 200. Because of this and the fact that she had had both herpes zoster and esophogeal candidiasis, she was officially diagnosed with AIDS. The doctor had said she was in the final stage of the disease; she should start to prepare herself and her family in case she could no longer live alone and take care of herself. Cindy had watched many friends and acquaintances die from AIDS over the past ten years. She had been able to put off the fact that it would someday happen to her, too. But when she was diagnosed, the reality shock sent Cindy spinning into a binge of tranquilizers and cocaine followed by a severe depression. She had felt incapable of preparing herself a meal, never mind preparing her family for her death.

During these months, Cindy developed a habit of mixing her pills together in a jar on the end table next to her favorite chair. She recognized them by their various colors and shapes. And, actually, it did not matter if she were to confuse them because she rarely took them. Usually she needed all her energy to force herself out of bed to get to the methadone program. She thought of little except returning home to bed. She ate a meal if someone brought food. Otherwise she lived on cereal (if she had milk) and canned soup. She showered when her hair felt stringy. She took whatever was offered to get numb rather than to get high. She lost forty-eight pounds; her face looked drawn and skeletal. She soon began to look as if she had advanced AIDS.

Cindy had graduated from college at age twenty-one with a degree in English. She had been quiet in school, but recalled many happy days and weekend nights with her group of friends. She had not made many friends in college, and tried hard to fit in with the few she had. She especially dreaded evenings alone. She had simply tried to pass the courses and to avoid dealing with the stress of approaching adulthood. She had developed a high tolerance for alcohol during her long evenings. This made it easy to agree to the occasional weekend binges where someone always showed up with marijuana. This was when she found that she could get the same high without the hangover.

After graduation she missed those occasional weekends. She watched her old high school friends return home and get jobs after their college years. Most seemed to have boyfriends and dreamy plans. Cindy felt isolated. She found that her degree did not lead into any career. Soon most of her friends were busy with their new lives.

When she ran into a college buddy, they reminisced about the wild parties they had survived. She began to think that those years were not so bad. They decided to get together the coming Friday night. Not only was the marijuana plentiful, but there were pills and cocaine. The leap to IV drug use was not planned.

Cindy's memories of these years were vague and unpleasant. She had a distinct memory of waking up in the emergency room one morning. She was told she had been found unconscious in the park. Her clothes were torn, and her arms and body were covered with bruises. Having no recollection of the previous evening was frightening for her. That was when she began the methadone program. Although it helped to reduce the drug craving, she still had binges of cocaine use when any stressful situation arose.

Fluctuating between 120 and 160 pounds, often within a matter of weeks reduced the tone of Cindy's muscles and skin. When her weight dropped, her doctor had prescribed an appetite stimulant such as Megace, which caused a craving for any type of food. This resulted in a buildup of subcutaneous fat. When she relapsed, she neither ate nor slept. She rapidly developed an emaciated look around her cheeks and eyes. Combined with the atrophy of muscles from an inactive, sedentary lifestyle, it gave her a look she dreaded.

But today, as she glanced at the clock, and briefly shut her eyes, she knew she would not have that uncontrollable urge to use. She knew because she had a plan. Her day was going to include the usual methadone dosing, checking out the neighborhood, a big breakfast, and seeing several new acquaintances at a Narcotics Anonymous meeting. Of course, she also would fit in the continuous medication regime which required that she remember to take a total of twenty-one pills a day at five different times. She was used to this by now; it had become a minor annoyance rather than a chore. When she began it, Cindy had been skeptical of the benefits of such a complicated regimen. She had been fearful of the side effects, both known and unknown. It was not until two months later, when her viral load had dropped and her CD4+ count had risen to the level of a year before, that she became committed to the treatment.

With the development of protease inhibitors and the dramatic and promising research into prolonging life for PLWA, Cindy had been forced to think about the future. Her initial reaction was elation at the change in her life expectancy. Within a few days, however, she became more thoughtful. She had spent the previous two years in a vacuum. Planning for the future had not been an option. Depression had allowed her to neglect and abuse her health. She had become dependent on Social Security as her only source of income.

After a month on the new therapy, her doctor had beamed when he shared the results of her latest blood work. Since taking the triple combination including a protease inhibitor, her CD4+ count had risen to 192. Cindy had commented at the time, "If I had known I would live this long, I would have taken better care of myself." He had responded that she could live a very long time as things looked at that point, and that it was never too late to work at being healthy.

At the urging of her nurse case manager, Cindy began to think about ways to begin to become more active. The last of the snow had melted, marking the beginning of spring. A spring morning seemed an appropriate time to begin a new outlook on life. After receiving her daily methadone dose, Cindy returned home, as usual, but instead of going directly inside and lying down, she sat on the step of her building. This was difficult for her to do because, always being concerned about the opinions of others, she was self-conscious about her daily trip to the program. She forced herself to stay there for five minutes, observing the coming and going of people and traffic. It was that day that for the first time she noticed the yellow and white crocuses someone had planted to the side of the step. She marveled that such delicate and beautiful living things could persist year after year. It occurred to her that her own life had followed a similar course of good times and hardship. In fact, she could relate to the repetitive pattern of starting out, tentatively emerging, only to once again succumb to stress and then relapse in drug use. Instead of being buried under the snow, she had hidden under her bedcovers as she settled in to accumulate the necessary forces to once again emerge in recovery.

Buoyed by this communion with nature, Cindy was able to repeat her vigil on the stoop for the next several mornings. She considered whether she would be able to walk as far as the corner. On Saturday she attempted to walk to the small playground four blocks away. Cindy walked to the corner and peered down the street to see how many children were on the swings and slides. Encouraged by the fact that there were only two or three at this early hour, she began to walk. Once again she was amazed at the number of small gardens and trees with spring buds, which she had never noticed as she drove by several times a day. On Sunday, she sat on the park bench at the edge of the playground for several minutes, enjoying the cool breeze and the cloudless sky.

Cindy soon began looking forward to her brief outings. She dug out an old umbrella on one drizzly morning. She bundled up in a sweatshirt under her jacket on cooler mornings. While she would return directly home and resume the normal pattern of her days, these outings, like spring and like her hope for the future, were brand-new to her.

As her legs became accustomed to the activity, Cindy felt the need to use other muscles. She asked around about other activities and soon found herself at the community center. The swimming, tennis, and aerobics did not interest her. When she saw three older women strolling by, swinging their arms, she was immediately curious about their group. She signed up for the mile-long walk, which left from the center three mornings a week. The time fit well into her other commitments such as the methadone program and clinic appointments.

By the time summer rolled in, Cindy was surprised that she felt hungry in the mornings after her walks. She had a long-standing once-a-day eating habit, then snacking on candy or junk food in the late afternoon. When a cooking class was announced at the health clinic, Cindy surprised herself by volunteering to join. A dietitian offered nutritional counseling and recipes to supplement and coordinate with the new cooking techniques. Cindy's thoughts no longer focused on her daily dosages, her overwhelming medication regime, and her desire to be a recluse. While still a loner, she was actively participating in multiple activities.

During periods of recovery, Cindy had been able to support herself. When she was diagnosed with AIDS, she qualified for disability. She knew she now needed to continue the state support for health care coverage and medication. Years before, Cindy had successfully completed a course in bartending and obtained a license, but was unable to successfully mix alcohol and any serious responsibilities. She had occasionally worked as a checkout clerk and as a waitress in a doughnut shop. Her favorite job had been in a bookstore. The pace was manageable and the store atmosphere was peaceful. Each attempt at employment, however, had ended when she had scraped together a little money and could not resist the craving for drugs. She decided to apply to a new bookstore that had recently opened several blocks from her apartment. She hoped to be able to increase her exercise routine by walking to and from work. Although the six to eight hours a week she was offered would not provide much more than pocket money, she accepted, knowing that she might have days when even this would be too much for her to work at this point.

Becoming bored with her routine, she bought a notebook and several pencils and began to record her daily activities. She elaborated on basic entries by describing some of the other people she met and parts of their conversations. When she began to jot down some of her reactions, she realized she was writing a journal just as she had been forced to do in college. Although she had hated the activity at that time, she now looked forward to it.

After filling several notebooks over the next month, Cindy shared what she had been doing with her nurse case manager, Nancy, who smiled, went to her car, and produced the most recently published edition of the local AIDS chapter newsletter. The first article on the first page was about the exciting numbers of individuals who were submitting poetry, letters, and short articles about their newfound energies. Cindy shyly produced several of her own pieces. Impressed, Nancy offered to bring them to the editor of the newsletter for his review. Cindy agreed as long as she remained anonymous. When one was published in the next edition, Cindy felt as if she had found another reason to continue to fight, and that the daily battle was worth the effort.

As her stamina increases, Cindy has been able to volunteer at the local AIDS chapter. Her life has been turned around. While it is heart wrenching to see others fail, unable to tolerate the new treatments, she finds support among her new group of friends and draws strength from her newfound ability to reach out to others.

LESSON 10: DEALING WITH THE CHANGE
IN EXPECTATIONS

With the development of medications, treatments, and improved diagnostics, the face of AIDS is changing. Short-term goals are being replaced by long-term expectations. This presents a challenge to health care providers in terms of offering optimal treatment options. It also comes as a surprise to patients who, up till recently, have been living their lives believing that their future is *now*.

Health care management considerations include choosing among various combinations of available pharmaceutical products, deciding when to initiate therapy, and evaluating the response to treatment. The challenge is to tailor treatment to each patient. An ideal result is a rise in the CD4+ count and a decrease in the viral load. Of particular value is to monitor the plasma HIV ribonucleic acid (or viral load) because substantial suppression can occur within a matter of days. The CD4+ count response is more gradual, requiring up to three months to reflect the effectiveness of therapy. Investigators from the Multicenter AIDS Cohort Study over a nine-year period have shown the value of the combination of CD4+ count/viral load measurement as a predictor of disease progression. Used routinely, these measurements are invaluable for the assessment of treatment efficacy and to predict clinical failure (Mellors et al., 1996).

Scientists have found that combination therapy which includes protease inhibitors can delay disease progression by interfering with reproduction of the HIV virus. The Centers for Disease Control and Prevention have reported that there has been a decline in the number of deaths from AIDS since early in 1995, when AIDS was the leading cause of death for Americans aged twenty-five to forty-four. The fact that life expectancy for AIDS patients has doubled can be attributed to the implementation of new therapies and treatment options (Statlanders, 1997).

There are both ethical and economic concerns about treatment with protease inhibitors, nucleosides and nonnucleoside reverse transcriptase inhibitors, and antiretrovirals. These include medication adherence, cost, cost savings, long-term side effects, and quality of life.

Strict adherence to the prescribed regime is essential for both successful outcome and to avoid the development of drug-resistant strains of the virus. This typically means a patient must take a variety of medications according to a strict schedule each day. For best absorption, it is specified whether most of these drugs should be taken with or without food. Due to a low percentage of bioavailability per tablet, some require that two to three tablets be taken two to three times per day. This results in the need to develop and follow a schedule of when to wake, eat, and go back to sleep based on medication administration times. This is difficult at best even for individuals who are used to following such a demanding and restrictive routine. Creative ways of reminding and motivating others are being studied.

Although the cost of combination drug therapy is significantly higher than previous medication regimes, the fact that their use has reduced overall treatment costs provides incentive for continued research. Cost savings are related to the fact that by controlling the viral load, the immune system is able to actively resist opportunistic infections. This translates into decreased use of costly interventions such as hospitalizations, intravenous medications or parenteral nutrition, and referrals to specialists.

Due to rapid development and Federal Drug Administration approval, to date there has been no opportunity to research the long-term side effects of these medications. Health care practitioners need to follow the literature for updated information in order to be knowledgeable about newly discovered interactions and implications for treatment.

Quality of life is best promoted by understanding the needs and goals of the individual. Through the open sharing of information about treatment risks, benefits, and impact on daily living, the patient will be able to make an informed decision.

Ethical considerations encompass all these issues. Each individual will identify quality of life in a different way. Society and the health care system as a whole are affected by the potential for the development of resistant strains of HIV if medication adherence is not possible. While current analysis indicates that preventive interventions are significantly less costly than the treatment of active, opportunistic infections, research is still ongoing. While preliminary research clearly indicates the benefits of protease inhibitors, patients need to be informed that the long-term effects remain to be seen. Because of the sheer number of pills that need to be taken as scheduled as well as the potentially debilitating side effects, some may not welcome combination therapy. Through active treatment planning and mutually established goals, the patient and the health care practitioner are preparing today for the unpredictable future.

PART III:
MANAGING THE HOSPICE
PHASE AT HOME

Chapter 11

"Will You Still Love Me?"

Leslie opened the door for the initial home visit with the remark, "What are you here for?" After the nurse introduced herself and explained what a visiting nurse's role could be, Leslie responded loudly, "Then get me some medicine because I am sick!" Leslie was forty-one, a former secretary, and a mother of four children. Her older son and daughter lived in their own apartments in a nearby area. Her eleven- and three-year-old sons lived with her. She was connected to a case manager for help with care of the children, shopping, transportation, and budgeting. Her case manager had been following Leslie for about two years now and had vouched for her being a warm-hearted woman. This was demonstrated by the decorations around the otherwise simple apartment.

Leslie had been discharged from the hospital two weeks earlier with a diagnosis of bacterial pneumonia. In addition, she suffered from wasting syndrome, chronic headaches, and inner ear inflammation. Her CD4+ count was 10. The ear infection had severely impaired her hearing. As a result, she felt the need to shout, and others needed to speak even more loudly back to her. On the day of the first visit, she had finished the prescribed course of erythromycin and was having recurrent productive cough, fever, and shortness of breath. It was obvious that she needed medical as well as nursing intervention. Efforts to persuade her to make a same-day appointment at the clinic where a nurse practitioner could assess these symptoms were unsuccessful. From past experience she knew that clinic visits in this condition often resulted in hospitalization.

"I'm not leaving this house so close to Christmas!" she shouted. "Can't you see I am all ready and I have spent everything on this Christmas?"

It was a week before Christmas. She had a large, pretty tree surrounded by many packages. Her highly energetic three-year-old continually interrupted with requests for attention. It was easy to understand why she wished to be at home.

Leslie had a reputation for missing clinic appointments. Her physician also was well aware of her attitude of defiance. Unfortunately, she had a fever of 102 degrees and a hacking cough. Her physician reluctantly agreed by telephone to oral antibiotics, decongestants, and a bronchodilating inhaler based on a promise by Leslie to keep a clinic appointment after the holidays. However, as Leslie responded positively to this course of therapy, she demanded that the doctors continue to treat her by phone. This resulted in an impasse since repeatedly prescribing medication without physically assessing the patient contradicted the clinic's policy. Although she did go to the clinic three times over the course of the next eight months, she remained unpredictable about follow-up.

Leslie had denied her risk for HIV infection and was diagnosed with full-blown AIDS three years before. At the same time her youngest son was also diagnosed as HIV positive.

She had overcome her drug addiction when she discovered she was pregnant. She continued to withhold the diagnosis from her family and friends. For the first time in her life, she had achieved stability and physical comfort. With the help of her case manager, she had an apartment, custody of her children, and food in the refrigerator. She could respect herself. She had control over her daily decisions. She was seeking the respect of others and control over her fears. To do this she had to be able to trust enough to share her emotional as well as physical needs. It was vital that Leslie be allowed to set the pace for developing that trust within her relationship with the home care team.

The nursing care plan goals were to provide early intervention with the recurrent respiratory and sinus infection, and to provide education on the importance of nutrition and medication adherence. Leslie was referred to the medical social worker to work on relapse prevention. Assessments were ongoing for the need to refer to a home health aide for personal care, a volunteer for companionship and transportation, and a chaplain for spiritual counseling.

The nurse visited once a week to do a physical assessment and fill her pill pack. Often the pills were untouched from week to week. It is important for the home care nurse to know what the patient is actually doing with medications. By gaining permission to fill and monitor the pill pack, it is possible to understand changes in health status. The fact that Leslie was not taking these medications was significant because it meant more vigilance was needed in checking for symptoms of opportunistic infection.

Out of respect for the patient's privacy, home visits are scheduled in advance, and every effort is made to keep them. However, because Leslie had no telephone, team members had to drop by unannounced. Occasionally Leslie would be found intoxicated and the house in disarray. To her credit, she had always made alternative arrangements for the children on these days. She would politely ask that the worker come back the next day and, if possible, the worker would oblige.

Leslie was not necessarily happy with her choices. Whether she had other alternatives or not, she seemed to make decisions based on her driving need to be in control of her situation. To establish a mutually trusting relationship, it is equally important that people be offered options for treatment and intervention and that their choices be respected. She also was not shy about making her opinions known. One of the most frequent offers of help was a home health aide: "Leslie, a home health aide could help with the laundry and start a meal for you and the boys." In the spirit of negotiation, it would be suggested, "We could start with only one or two afternoons a week to see how it would work out." Her reply inevitably would be, "I don't want any strangers in this house. I already got more people in here than I can deal with!" Or more honestly, "I don't always do what I am supposed to be doing, or go where I am supposed to be going, and I don't want no one to be here watching me."

She eventually agreed to a home health aide when her shortness of breath limited climbing the stairs to her bedroom to only once a day. With the kitchen, bathroom, and laundry facilities on the first level, she needed to conserve energy for getting around the apartment.

It was particularly difficult to accept her choice about not going to the clinic. When her physician insisted on seeing her before reordering any prescriptions, if she did not go, she had no prophylaxis for opportunistic infections. Leslie did not seem to give this much thought. Knowing that one aspect of her health that had consistently responded to medication was her chronic respiratory condition, the nurse would point out, "If you do not want to go to the clinic, you need to know it means you will not get an antibiotic for your cough." Leslie stubbornly refused, saying, "I am too sick to be waiting around in that place! I need to stay home and rest!"

The nurse could only reconfirm the offer, saying, "Leslie, remember that when you are ready to go to the clinic, we can make the appointment."

Building trust seemed to be a process that was never complete. Leslie might reach out to someone who offered assistance, but the effort was motivated by *her* perception of what she needed. She had no faith in the opinion of any home health care worker. She had no need to play the game of trying to befriend or please. She did test the nurse's commitment to her on two occasions, however. During a long wait in the clinic, she was offered a mint. She immediately asked if she could have the whole package. The next time the nurse was in her home, the package of mints was sitting untouched on the side table. Leslie had been testing the nurse's reaction. She needed to know if her request would be valued. The nurse felt she needed to send the message that she did regard and respect her as an individual.

One day Leslie discussed her difficulty of not being able to get in touch with a friend because she was too weak to walk to the telephone booth. She was offered a ride for the short block. No sooner was she back in the car than she asked, "Could I have some change for cigarettes?"

The standard response to all requests for money was given. "Leslie, I would rather give you something else."

"But, I want a cigarette!"

"You know, Leslie, you have a lot of trouble breathing. I am not going to give you money for cigarettes."

"You can't tell me what to do! I'll just go get some money somewhere else!"

She sat there venting for a few more minutes before the nurse said, "How about if we go get a cup of coffee?"

"No! I want a cigarette!"

After driving home in silence, they went into the house, where Leslie turned and said, "How about going for coffee?"

Having experienced frequent disappointment and repeated rejection, she no longer had the ability to trust anyone. To gain Leslie's cooperation, the nurse needed to prove repeatedly that she and Leslie had the same goals. In a situation such as this, mutual respect is as close as a relationship gets to a level of trust.

It wasn't until Leslie had lost an additional twenty pounds that she agreed to have help in her home. Until that time, Leslie had faithfully kept both boys fed and dressed. She insisted her older son attend school regularly, even though he would have been of help to her in watching and disciplining his younger brother. She was strict and forceful, but always appeared to be fair. As her health failed, the case manager was able to coordinate custody of her eleven-year-old son with his father. Her youngest son was spending most days and nights in the nursery for families with AIDS. Both children received education and support from this agency. Although she could barely walk up the stairs, Leslie limited the agreement for home health aide services to every other day for assistance with meals and laundry only. This was two short weeks before she died.

Leslie was family-oriented, but that did not necessarily mean she got along with her family. Although her sister and her only daughter lived within a few blocks of her apartment, she would have to cry and cajole them to come over to help her. However, no sooner would they walk in the door than she would scream and berate them either for not coming sooner or for not performing tasks according to her standards. This behavior would then drive them away once again. The rest of her family lived several hundred miles away. Although she sincerely wanted her mother to come to be with her, in the past visits and telephone calls were marked by angry words and demands. Nevertheless she named her mother as heir and guardian of her children. Her case manager had spent many hours coordinating and finalizing the documents to ensure that Leslie's wishes were documented and that Leslie's mother agreed to honor those wishes. One of the goals that we were able to accomplish was to legalize a living will and durable power of attorney which named her mother as her agent. Through telephone conversations, the medical social worker and case manager were able to ensure that her mother understood the implications of the documents. It was important that she know exactly what type of care Leslie wished to receive from health care workers either at home or in a hospital setting in the event that she would be unable to speak for herself.

Several weeks before the dramatic decline in her stamina, Leslie seemed to be anticipating the inevitable. She became centered around both her appearance and her mother's arrival. One day she showed the nurse a pretty, ruffled, black dress covered with colored bows.

"What do you think of this dress?" she asked.

The nurse smiled because it looked so different from her usual outfits. "It is very pretty, Leslie. Where do you plan to wear it?"

"I want to look nice for my mother. She is coming next week. Do you think we could dye it all black?"

"I don't see why not. I think it would look very nice like that."

She had a pair of black high-heeled shoes that needed a little repair. When she had fixed up her outfit, she seemed satisfied.

On the day after her mother arrived, Leslie asked for a priest. It took several days to coordinate the actual home visit. In the meantime, she asked both her sister and the nurse to read her excerpts from her Bible. She died the day after she received the priest's blessing.

Leslie dealt with her losses by striking out at those who she knew were least likely to abandon her. She never blamed others for her illness, yet her anger was very close to the surface, and it seemed to obstruct her peace of mind. At the same time, this anger fueled her courage to continue the daily struggle to maintain dignity. She intensely wanted to die with dignity in her own home.

The ability to have choices gave Leslie the control she needed to overcome her fears. PLWA fear dementia, physical pain, and disfigurement, and, most of all, dying alone. According to our care plan goals, she was able to remain safely in her own home, at an optimal level of function. Choices were continually offered. To meet individual needs, it had to be clear that choices were limited to time or place. Communication amongst her physician, case manager, and family were facilitated. Case management, communication, and compassion were vital to meeting Leslie's needs.

In spite of different perceptions of these needs, cooperation was possible because each team member understood and adhered to the boundaries of their disciplines. Being in control of her immediate surroundings gave Leslie the ability to focus on improving her present situation rather than brooding on the disappointments she had experienced. By controlling her surroundings she was able to control her fears. She maintained direction over some of the circumstances of her death by completing the tasks most important to her dignity. She maintained herself and her two younger children independently within her own home up until the final weeks of her life. She created an image of responsibility and courage. By reaching out to her family she expressed her love for them to the best of her ability. Because of this she is remembered positively, for her strengths, rather than for her failures.

LESSON 11: STAYING FOCUSED

A vital component of the home care nurse's care plan is to work toward mutual goals. Early on this may seem easy. Just as in home construction, the laying of the foundation and setting up of the skeleton-like walls moves along rapidly. Meeting needs for food and shelter, acute symptom relief, and home care equipment are only the basics. After addressing the immediate psychosocial needs, the painstakingly slow part is discovering successful interventions to keep the patient and family safe.

There are typically many issues to address on that first day: nutrition supplements, contacting the doctor for prescriptions, making clinic appointments, ordering medical equipment, setting up a pill pack, teaching home safety and hygiene, and referral to other community agencies. However, it is the way that first problem on that first day is handled that reassures the patient and caregiver of the nurse's and the home health agency's commitment to helping as much and as quickly as possible. It is from this point that the work toward long-term solutions begins.

It is not difficult to recognize an individual's needs; they are usually obvious. However, the right solution is not always so obvious. Sometimes there are "quickie" solutions: Out of food this week? Well, let me run to the emergency food cupboard at the office. No way to get to the clinic/the bank/the methadone program? Well, just this once, I'll give you a ride. Need a loaf of bread? Well, I'll loan you two dollars. You didn't have lunch yet? Well, let's go across the street—my treat. Need that prescription filled? Come on, let's go to the pharmacy together.

While these innocent, small acts of kindness are offered with the best intentions, they can result in disaster. If there is no money for food because of active substance use, that is the subject that must be addressed. Usually errands are run by the patient's support network. If there is a breakdown in that network, it needs attention. The need for companionship or conversation may be a cry for attention or a more serious problem. Neglect to fill a prescription may be a sign of dementia or an attempt to use the nurse as an agent to refill a prescription before it is actually due.

Finding long-term rather than Band-Aid solutions is hard work. It means multiple phone calls to agencies responsible for specific services. It means tedious coordination of all services. It means communication of the plan and the outcome of interventions to the primary MD or clinic. It means team conferences on difficult problems. It means educating a community as well as families and caregivers about the patient's needs. Perhaps most difficult of all, it means saying "no" to the very person with whom we are trying to connect and build a trusting relationship.

The desire to give a patient a gift is based on ordinary human compassion and the health care worker's ability to provide that gift. However, to impulsively respond to a need for an item or a service may send the wrong message. If the responsibilities of the medical social worker, nurse, home health aide, and volunteer overlap, it can confuse the team, the patient, and result in inefficient delivery of care. If one member of the team gives food or money, it undermines the services of other members of the team. Priorities must be mutually agreed upon. Each home care agency should have a set of guidelines for continuity among health care providers.

By differentiating between the roles of friend and professional, we enable the patient and family to help themselves. Education about food resources, budgeting, alcohol or narcotic anonymous groups, support groups, psychiatric or psychological counseling services, or community ride programs can and do save home health care workers from becoming overwhelmed and from neglecting other responsibilities to this and other patients.

Chapter 12

"Why Don't I Die?"

Richard spent the last eighteen months of his life in the only safe place he could find: his own bed. His physician referred Richard to hospice because he saw rapidly advancing physical deterioration in the form of septic sinusitis, recurrent bronchitis, pneumonia, and oral thrush. His CD4+ count was less than 50. Richard said that he knew he was dying and that he accepted this as inevitable. He was only thirty-eight. His cold, detached demeanor challenged anyone to question his judgment or opinion or any matter. Having spent twelve of his twenty-three adult years in jail, he was accustomed to confinement and resigned to his bleak future. He said he could recall the very day he shared an infected syringe and contracted HIV six years before.

Because Richard said his greatest problem was peripheral neuropathy in both lower feet and legs, we agreed that this should be our priority in developing a plan of care. He also reported intermittent but severe headaches. Within a few weeks we had addressed these comfort needs. Since he had been receiving Percocet (oxycodone) with little relief, low dose M S Contin (controlled-release morphine) was tried. Because of a history of anxiety, he was prescribed diazepam three times a day. As a combination treatment for depression and the neuropathy, he began Elavil (amitriptyline) at bedtime. His decision to continue prophylaxis with dapsone and Diflucan (fluconazole) was supported.

Within several more weeks, it was apparent that he was taking more medication than the amounts prescribed. With comfort still as our goal, we requested prescriptions to meet what Richard seemed to need to deal with the physical discomfort. The M S Contin was reassessed every two weeks, but because of nausea, he was inconsistent in dosing. After four months of juggling dosages, it was decided to add codeine every four hours as needed for headaches, and within a few weeks Richard chose to stop the M S Contin completely. By this time the Elavil dose was increased significantly. He followed this regime with more consistency and was able to function in his apartment with minimal assistance. Over the next year, both the codeine and the Elavil were gradually increased, while the other drugs used remained constant.

His two-room, second-floor apartment with a kitchenette seemed cramped because he was using the front room as a bedroom. Plopped in the middle of the room was a full-size mattress, which he and his girlfriend and primary caregiver, Anne, shared. His physical environment was difficult to appreciate for several reasons. He was averse to daily showers and he spent most of his days as well as nights lying on the mattress on the floor, chain smoking. In addition to the mattress, there was only enough room for one upholstered chair. The small back room was furnished with a couch and a rocking chair. It also was needed for storage of clothing and other accumulated items. Although this room would have been more appropriate, the assessment visits were rarely conducted there. Typically, Richard was lying in bed, and Anne sat in the chair. The only place left for the German shepherd, nurse, and any visitors to sit was the foot of his mattress.

On the nurse's arrival, Richard was usually lying on top of the covers with his eyes closed. Typically, a few minutes were spent greeting first the dog and then Anne, who conscientiously kept the team updated on all variations in his behavior or condition. Richard would then acknowledge the nurse's presence. While this was sometimes done voluntarily, he occasionally would speak only if spoken to directly. Thirty to forty-five minutes of general conversation seemed to be necessary before he would discuss what was going on with his respiratory, digestive, or neuromuscular status. This would be followed by the evaluation of vital signs, a general physical assessment, and any necessary phone calls to the physician or pharmacy. The time spent with Anne discussing events in their lives and his response to variations in treatment seemed to be needed as an introduction to the intimate aspects of his life. Richard needed someone to read between the lines and anticipate his needs. He needed an advocate for his safety and comfort because he was unable to admit that he had any needs at all.

The depth of Richard's emotional pain and depression were not discovered until a pattern of physical changes was recognized as coinciding with his monthly medication delivery. On a regular, monthly basis he temporarily suffered severe, increased weakness, vomiting, and changes in mental status. The first pill count was done during a period when Richard was too sick to object. It was found that he had taken approximately one-third of his month's supply of diazepam and Elavil in two days. He still had enough dapsone and fluconazole to last several months. Richard was given an ultimatum: for prescriptions to continue, he had to consent to let his girlfriend control his medications on a weekly delivery basis from one pharmacy. This was extremely difficult for Richard to accept. As his disease progressed, his motivation to remain in charge never lessened. He needed to control every aspect of his very limited lifestyle. His jail-bred habits of hiding contraband under his mattress (a jackknife, a screwdriver, pens), denying himself simple pleasures (going out of doors, spending time with friends or relatives), and never volunteering any information seemed to increase. It would be an exaggeration to say that anyone ever had a real conversation with Richard, because he said so little. Occasionally, he did silently share a book of poems or a portfolio of artwork he had done in prison.

"These are beautiful, Richard." His sharing was a way of communicating.

"Yeah, I guess so," was his response. His verbal replies were terse.

"It's very impressive. You give a lot to others by sharing these."

All he would or could respond was, "Yeah. I tried." He knew his limitation, but, he also new his ability to write a poem or draw a picture communicated more of his inner feelings than he had ever been able to convey through conversation.

Following his release from prison, he had connected with the state AIDS education center. He had once been invited to speak at a local community college about his experience with AIDS, and he was obviously proud of the newspaper article that praised his effort.

His usual silence was countered by the fact that he did everything else he enjoyed to excess: eating several pizzas at one sitting, drinking gallons of soda, sleeping for days, chain smoking all the cigarettes available. Perhaps these behaviors also related to his years of self-denial. Knowing this, however, did not make life any easier for Anne, who had seen him through the unpleasant side effects of repeated overdoses. Although he maintained a quiet demeanor during nursing visits, she described temper tantrums and verbal abuse. Even though he was weak, she needed to watch her purse. Her commitment came from the depths of her heart and she stubbornly intended to have closure with the relationship.

As the months passed, his messy corner became a sad joke. Yet, it was important to respect it. As it became more and more difficult for him to get up from floor level, it also became more difficult for others to deal with bathing, feeding, and occasional incontinence. A hospital bed would have made life easier. He passively listened to the explanation of the advantages of posture and position changes, as well as the ease of getting out of bed to go to the bathroom. He closed his eyes when it was explained how proper body mechanics for lifting and turning him could make life easier for others. The problem was that Anne shared the full-size mattress on the floor. Changing this arrangement would mean she would have to sleep in the back room.

It was only when the nurse picked up the telephone to put in the request for the hospital bed that Richard revealed a glimpse of his true vulnerability by tearfully asking Anne, "Can I come visit you once in a while?" She decided to continue with the current situation. She had been loyal to him through many long months, following several years of a difficult, abusive relationship. At this point they both needed to close the relationship in a positive way.

It wasn't until Richard had been visited once or twice a week for a year that he asked, "Why don't I die?" This expression of normal emotion was the first the nurse had witnessed.

The nurse responded, "I don't know, Richard. Can you tell me?"

He answered, "I don't know."

Trying to continue this breakthrough, the nurse asked him, "What part of your routine do you find the most difficult?"

He answered with a well-worn phrase. "There is nothing to do. Not here. Not in this city, and not in this state." Thereafter, he repeated his question many times, but it became rhetorical; he never wanted to pursue the answer. Once he told a story about going out of the apartment, alone, and crossing the street to the cemetery. In his current physical state it was highly unlikely that he had been able to negotiate the winding stairs and safely cross the heavily traveled street. However, he said, "I woke up holding onto and swinging from the gate." The entrance to the cemetery did, indeed, have large, heavy, metal gates. "Now," he said, "I am thinking about swinging on the gates of Hell." Once, very calmly, he said, "Gone but not forgotten. That would be good."

It was during this period that Richard began to look at his mortality and his life. This was the turning point at which he could choose to help others help him. By acknowledging and validating his feelings, his relationship with his health care team and his primary care giver could develop. It was during this time that he relinquished control over his medication. When he stopped the binging on tranquilizers and narcotics, the episodes of gastrointestinal upsets and extreme mood swings also diminished.

The medical social worker was actively involved in the coordination of legal documents to delegate both a power of attorney and an agent for the durable power of attorney. This team member was also available for funeral arrangements in the weeks prior to Richard's death. Addressing these issues in advance gave Richard the opportunity to express his wishes, relieving Anne of total responsibility. Although Richard would never discuss his funeral with any team member, Anne was able to discuss his wishes with him during opportune moments. Because the team gave her the support she needed, she was able to follow through on the necessary arrangements. She was given durable power of attorney, and both she and Richard felt comfortable about their commitment to his wishes to avoid medical or life-support interventions. The funeral arrangements were made well in advance of his death, easing the need for decisions during the first days of bereavement.

Richard was visited by a chaplain every other week. He also had a volunteer who came in weekly. A home health aide was accepted only when he could no longer get to the bathroom or the refrigerator without assistance. Richard was a white, self-proclaimed bigot with a tough-guy image. Damon, the home health aide assigned, was a tall, muscular, black, rehabilitated alcoholic with a heart of gold.

Although Richard refused to speak to Damon for the first week or so, they did eventually become the best of friends.

Richard was allowed the dignity of deciding almost every aspect of his care in his own home, at his own level of comfort. The only dictated issues were related to safety. He backed off from soul-searching as quickly as he brought it up. He never said thank you. He expressed his satisfaction by allowing others to come to him. He eventually expressed his trust by sharing his poetry and drawings done in prison. He died peacefully, among those he loved.

Anne, as primary caregiver, was able to realize her desire to keep Richard at home because of the physical help from the home health aide, the respite offered by the volunteers, the spiritual support from the chaplain, and the emotional support and education from the professional nurse, social worker, and hospice physician. The team was consistently available to address changes in his condition and creatively mold a plan of care to meet their needs.

The care plan for Richard centered around his need for control. His fear of loneliness and humiliation were respected. The fact that he trusted only those who allowed him to maintain his sense of dignity was recognized. By bargaining, a balance was found between the need to maintain home safety with his desire for control: if he cut down on smoking, he could increase the diazepam, and if he allowed Anne to administer his medications, the doses could be increased; he could choose a change in either dosage or frequency. Choices were consistently and regularly offered and his decisions were accepted. Interventions were continually reevaluated to ensure that the team was on track toward the goals of safety and comfort. Promises were kept. Richard and his situation were assessed through his own eyes in order to meet his needs.

LESSON 12: RECOGNIZING THE TURNING POINT

In working with a population with overwhelming need, priorities may seem obvious. However, they are sometimes less obvious to the individual who has learned to survive under extremely difficult and dangerous circumstances for many years. Some have been accustomed to extreme poverty. Some have spent years in prison. Most health care practitioners can only imagine these circumstances. It is necessary to empathize with the past to understand the present. By candidly and respectfully asking questions, the individual's expectations can be learned and a plan of care agreed on. By accepting the limitations, available home health care services can be presented effectively.

One inevitable component of working with an individual with AIDS is patience. The early weeks of establishing ground rules for the relationship require many hours of discussion with both the patient and other community agencies. The subsequent weeks or months spent together, however, are usually pleasant because they are less intense. During this time the home health care practitioner needs to remain focused on the goals. Goal setting involves continual evaluation and reevaluation of the patient's needs.

The advice must be the same every day, from every health care worker. Consistency will offer security and safety. No exceptions should be made. The patient and family should be contacted frequently and as scheduled. Follow-up should be prompt, courteous, and consistent.

The patient's residence is always where the patient is visited. This may mean visiting a temporary shelter, a group home, or a friend's or relative's house. This allows the patient to feel unthreatened and open to establishing a plan of care. Also, we need to evaluate the home environment for safety and individual functional level. It is in this relaxed atmosphere that the health care worker can offer services and the patient can accept or decline them. What is said may not be what the patient expects or wants to hear. Situational relief, medical appointments, or home assistance may take weeks to establish.

As long as people feel vulnerable, they are unlikely to expose themselves any further in any way. The creation of a safe environment and an honest relationship opens the door for further interventions. As the value of these interventions is recognized by the patient and significant others, the risks will decrease. Even goals as basic as symptom management and comfort require cooperation for effective communication and understanding. The pain in a person's story must be understood to address its source and treatment. This often means understanding the emotional as well as the physical pain. The message must be sent that this person is valued and respected. Successful interventions encourage trust. In turn there is reduced risk of harmful behaviors and relapse.

Although the nurse and the patient may come from very different environments or cultures, they will always have one common goal: to improve the current situation and the patient's quality of life. In home and hospice care, nurses can expect to see the stages of grieving intermingle with the stages of preparation for change. By remaining focused, those stages can be recognized and support can be provided.

Chapter 13

"I Hate Living Like This"
Does Not Mean "Help Me Die"

One of the most challenging cases was also the shortest. Sam was referred following a hospital admission for pneumonia. According to Peter, his primary caregiver, Sam was actually hospitalized following an episode in the backyard in which he had chased Peter, swinging a two-by-four board. Before Sam did any harm, however, he collapsed and Peter managed to call an ambulance. After a one-week stay he was sent home on Bactrim twice a day for the pneumonia and Haldol three times a day for behavior control.

Peter felt paternal toward Sam, who was fifteen years his junior. He had become Sam's spokesperson as well as his caregiver. Peter described in detail how they had met in the city twenty years before. Their paths had crossed repeatedly since. Finally, he said, Sam had shown up on his doorstep, homeless, six months previously. Peter was not surprised that Sam had AIDS. He knew that Sam's impulsive, rootless lifestyle among artists and musicians across the country, as well as his cavalier attitude toward drugs, put him at high risk for exposure to HIV/AIDS.

Three months previously, Peter confronted Sam about his weight loss and at regular doctor visits. When Sam revealed that he had advanced AIDS and that he probably only had a few months to live, Peter resolved to take care of him.

Both men wanted one thing: privacy. They were reluctant to share any information with anyone, but had reached the point of desperation. Peter was torn between wanting the best care for Sam, guidance for himself, and protection from public scrutiny.

Sam's mental state fluctuated between lucid and delirious. The fact that he could not manage his own hygiene was complicated by

his frequent bouts of diarrhea. Peter found the accidental incontinence extremely upsetting. Obtaining his doctor's permission for
Imodium was easy. Persuading Sam to take the medication was more
difficult. Ultimately it was a choice between wearing disposable under-
garments or taking the antidiarrheal medication. Because Sam's preferred attire was undershorts and nothing else, it was obvious if wore a
diaper. Sam soon agreed to take the medication.

Sam had a host of other problems. Oral and esophageal thrush
coated his tongue and palate so severely that he could hardly swallow. He had multiple prescriptions for antifungals, but he insisted
they did not help and refused to take them. His physician arranged
for him to have intravenous infusions of amphoteracin B in the
outpatient clinic. While the coordination of transportation and personal preparation was initially difficult, it was quickly recognized as
a positive change.

The decision to have outpatient treatment was made for two reasons. First, Sam's Medicare insurance did not fully cover home
intravenous infusion. Second, Peter was reluctant to take on the
responsibility of home infusion therapy in view of Sam's unpredictable behavior changes. Although the daily clinic treatments were
initially inconvenient, they were also a blessing. The time apart gave
an increasingly frazzled Peter some much-needed respite. Sam went
daily for three days with no notable progress. In fact the accumulation of exudate seemed worse. A strict regime of brushing three
times a day and rinsing with saline and nystatin swish-and-swallow
was started. It was negotiated that Sam could omit the swallow once
a day since he believed it upset his stomach. After three more days,
there was noticeable improvement in both Sam's appearance and the
amount of food he was eating comfortably. It was stressed that he
needed both topical and systemic treatment for continued relief of
the thrush. Apparently he agreed because he continued the regime.

This was not the case with the care of a superficial decubitus ulcer
on his coccyx, acquired during a hospital stay. It was washed daily
with peroxide and saline, a bio-occlusive dressing was applied, and an
explanation given regarding the need to leave it in place for the next
several days. Daily the nurse returned only to find he had removed it,
exposing the tender area to further irritation.

Sam was 6'1" and 130 pounds. His skin had a gray pallor and he paced the apartment continuously. He slept very little, day or night. Peter had to remember to give Sam Haldol (haloperidol) every eight hours without fail to obtain any cooperation with other medication, bathing, food, or rest.

For Sam's nutritional deficits, he was provided canned supplements. A quick review of his eating habits revealed that the convenience foods he normally ate were significantly low in protein and vitamins. A diet that would be easier to digest as well as high in protein and carbohydrates was recommended. Because it was low bulk, it also would help the diarrhea. By chilling and sipping the supplements he was able to take several cans a day.

Because of Sam's confusion, home safety needed to be addressed. Suggestions included locking the doors at night to keep Sam from leaving, writing emergency telephone numbers and posting them near the phone, preventing falls by positioning furniture for handholds throughout the house, and alerting local emergency agencies to the situation. Once boundaries were set, Sam's functional level improved. With consistent hygiene and mouth care he seemed more relaxed at home. Peter's comfort level with his responsibilities also increased with education about medication regimes and use of a pill pack as a reminder of the schedule. The situational depression both Sam and Peter felt improved as they saw these interventions making a difference.

Because of their diverse problems, Sam and Peter were ideal candidates for a multidisciplinary team. Such an approach benefits both the patient and the home health care worker. Typically, a primary nurse is assigned to each patient to do the majority of the home visits, and the team is kept up to date on all events during a weekly meeting. Additional nurses provide fresh insights and cover any time off. The medical social worker, chaplain, volunteer coordinator, on-call staff, and physician are called upon as needed. The mounting psychosocial and legal complications could not be dealt with by the primary nurse alone. This was explained to Peter in no uncertain terms. Despite their complex needs, both Sam and Peter adamantly refused to have any other team members involved. Not only did this limit their services, but it placed an unbalanced burden on the primary nurse. Repeated discussion of these limitations and the advantages of involving social services, a home health aide, and a spiritual counselor did not change their minds.

Sam's primary physician confirmed that he was indeed in the end stages of AIDs and that they had discussed his desire to have comfort measures only. Peter declared that he had both power of attorney and durable power of attorney, assuring the nurse that their lawyer had these documents, but he failed to ever produce them. Sam seemed eligible for state benefits to pay for medications, equipment, and supplies, but without proper applications, it was impossible to provide them. These were problems with which a nurse could empathize, but only a social worker could address effectively.

Both Peter and Sam spoke of the inevitable fact that Sam would die soon. Sam had lost his ability to concentrate on his longtime hobby of decoupage as well as the stamina to enjoy a music concert. He spoke of these losses with great regret and sadness. He did not like the way his life was ending. As many PLWA, he was suffering not only from social stigma, but also from a loss of friends and loss of sense of self, resulting in increasing isolation. Once, while Sam napped, Peter asked the nurse if she had heard of the Hemlock Society. He said he knew someone who was a member and was considering becoming a member. The nurse asked if Sam had expressed any intention or desire to end his life. Peter denied this, but went on to say that he knew Sam had loved his former life and that it was cruel to watch him slowly deteriorate. Finally, Peter asked if a bottle of morphine could be provided, in case Sam developed pain. The nurse assured Peter that Sam would receive any pain medication he needed, as it was needed, and that he would not suffer. However, it did not seem needed today.

One nurse was the only sounding board these two men had within their self-imposed boundaries. By relieving some physical discomfort, ordering equipment, and educating them about proper personal care and sanitary precautions, the nurse helped them to cope with Sam's physical disability. Also, they were able to free up the energy to grieve for these losses.

Sam was visited daily for the three weeks he was on the program. He often spoke of the fact that he was dying, but never did he ask about ways to hasten his death. He continued with the daily trips to the clinic for intravenous infusions because they provided some relief from the thrush. He denied being in any physical pain despite the wasting and diarrhea. He found he could rest easier in a hospital bed with an egg crate mattress than in his own waterbed. He accepted assurances that he would not suffer from pain and that Peter could have assistance from a home health aide to share any responsibilities for his personal care if he requested it. Peter assured him he would not die alone.

Sam rapidly became a shadow of the man he once was. He was fully aware of this fact and it was emotionally painful for him and for those around him. However, he sought relief, not escape, from his problems. Sympathy was not what he wanted, nor would it have helped as much as compassionate assessment and treatments which allowed him to die at home with dignity. There is literally a world of difference between saying "I hate living like this" and "Help me die."

LESSON 13: OPEN COMMUNICATION

The ability to listen and to discuss the most difficult of topics is the essence of communication. If a patient believes that the nurse is uncomfortable with certain topics, he or she may not bring them up a second time. Honesty in answering hard questions can be softened by offering hope through symptom management.

Fear of humiliation, loneliness, pain, and death are honest and universal emotions. While there is no formula or set of objective signs to predict just who will suffer emotionally, by expecting these as normal responses to tragic circumstances, the health care practitioner will be better prepared to deal with them. Internalizing these fears will result in anxiety or depression. Expressing these fears, raises the opportunity for alternative therapies.

Acknowledging depression and suicidal ideation should be a routine part of each assessment. These emotions are a normal part of anticipating grieving. Addressing the possible causes of a depression and actively seeking interventions to improve quality of life is part of the solution. Depression can result from pain or poor symptom management. It can also be exacerbated by drug side effects or interactions. Through communication with the primary physician it may be determined if a referral for psychotherapy or antidepressants is appropriate.

By asking, "What do you see as the worst problem today?" the patient is given the opportunity to share his or her perception of problems. This is important because the practitioner's assessment of the situation may be very different from that of the patient. The home health care practitioner may see a gaping need in the physical environment or in interpersonal relationships in the household, while these may be perfectly acceptable to the patient.

An individual's attitude toward the future affects the interpretation of suffering and illness. If someone believes that a treatment is inconvenient or uncomfortable for the moment, but there is relief in the future, he or she may wish to tolerate that discomfort. When hope for future treatments is exhausted, an increase in anxiety, depression, and the surfacing of suicidal thoughts can be expected. Reassurance of health care support is provided either within the home through the support network or by providing options in the community. This reassurance leads to choices other than premature end of life.

It is most appropriate that hospice address the issue of suicide prevention. Hospice workers specialize in relief from pain and suffering on the physical, emotional, and spiritual levels. It is by sharing patients' personal space, learning about their personal histories, and listening to their stories that the present needs can be understood. Through physical assessment and open communication among all members of the home care team, relief from persistent suffering can be provided. "The team's ultimate goal must not be merely to keep assisted suicide or euthanasia illegal, but rather to make them irrelevant!" (Byock, 1994, p. 8).

Chapter 14

Cliff-Hangers

To find Connie, you had to be an early bird. Her day actually started around 3 a.m. When the methadone would begin to wear off and she would awaken, restless, uncomfortable, and yearning for relief. She bounced back and forth between methadone maintenance programs, unable to keep up with the policies of any one for very long. When Connie was not seen for several days, we knew she had once again succumbed to a binge and could be found either in a local emergency unit or a jail. Occasionally she would call in response to a note left on her door or with a neighbor, but usually she waited in her apartment for one of us to find her. Not once did she call to complain or request crisis intervention. However, she knew we would come.

Connie had moved into a large public housing development just prior to admission to the home care program. The floors throughout the building were linoleum, and the walls were painted and bare. However, after living on the streets for the past several years, the two-room, sparsely furnished apartment was close to heaven on earth for Connie. She often slept on a folding mat in the front room, leaving the twin bed for one friend or another. Although she never admitted it, she seemed to long for the time she lived among friends on the streets. The food in the house usually consisted of leftovers from several meals sitting out on the stove near a pile of dirty dishes in the sink. Some mornings her speech would be somewhat slurred and deliberate, her hair soiled, and her clothing wrinkled. On these mornings she was reluctant to have a nurse visit. However, with some encouragement, she would come and sit on the couch, apologizing for the general state of the apartment or the other still-sleeping guests, while her medications were sorted out. Though the need for homemaking services was apparent, she was not eligible because she was not homebound.

It was not unusual to be greeted by a disheveled Connie matter-of-factly stating, "I took some diazepam yesterday. I just want you to know that."

A supportive response would be, "I appreciate your sharing that, Connie. You seem to feel bad about it."

"It makes me sleep all day and then I fall down and drop cigarettes, burning holes in the rug and things."

"So, you'd like to stop taking pills that do that to you?"

"Yeah, but when I'm around certain people, I can't help it."

Connie's living situation placed her among other substance users. They routinely traded or shared Valium (diazepam), Xanax (alprazolam), Percocet (oxycodone), and other prescription drugs. While it was known how and why Connie and her friends regularly got high, the success of any intervention depended upon her motivation to help herself. After she had been receiving visits for about six months, she revealed that she bought a prescription of diazepam monthly from a local doctor who regularly operated this sideline. By admitting this, she indicated her wish to stop. By obtaining a prescription from her regular doctor and gradually decreasing her dose weekly, she did stop buying prescriptions of diazepam. Occasionally she slipped into old habits by borrowing from friends, but she began to take a little better care of herself.

Connie's daily routine centered around the daily methadone dose. The methadone clinic opened at 6:00 a.m. Connie, like many others, usually arrived earlier. This daily ritual is followed seven days a week, 365 days a year, in sunny or stormy weather. These people are motivated by the desire to quench their drug hunger safely.

Connie was typical in that she would fall asleep in the late afternoon and awaken well before dawn. Although a blood test might have shown she still had a therapeutic level of methadone, it is the impending change in that level that the individual senses. She would wait anxiously for the next several hours until it was time to head over to the clinic.

Illegal drug use, sales, and related activities are not unusual at the programs, as the police are well aware. Neither was it unusual for Connie to be caught with illegal substances while socializing with friends. If she were arrested, she would not call. Connie's pride would not allow her to ask for help. A team effort was needed to support Connie through periods of relapse. Following one such incident the medical social worker interceded on her behalf by discussing her options for legal representation.

By missing meals, prescribed medication, and medical follow-up, Connie's PLWA's risk for opportunistic infections was increased. Other factors that contribute to health failure are stress and active substance use. She was monitored closely for weight and energy loss, bowel changes, skin changes, and increased incidence of pneumonia, sinusitis, thrush, and herpes.

Connie would be visited as prearranged on a weekly basis between 7:30 and 8:00 a.m. The first challenge would be to find and fill her pill pack according to the prescriptions available. This would be followed up with telephone verification to the clinic and/or pharmacy for those that were missing. If Connie lost her pill pack, it would be suggested that she look for it and the nurse would return the following day. Actually, she had two pill packs and each was often partially filled. By combining the leftover tablets, she was usually able to get through each week. The fact that her insurance benefit would not allow for lost medication meant she occasionally was between (and therefore without) prescriptions. This, too, had to be accepted as part of the risky lifestyle she led.

Connie would regularly attend the immunology/medical clinic. Her self-destructive behavior was offset by this demonstration of effort to maintain her fragile health. Her CD4+ count was below 50. She rarely kept up with the prescribed prophylaxis for opportunistic infections. Yet she truly intended to follow the doctor's directions week to week.

She would speak of her children only if directly asked. She stoutly declared, "I gave them birth. What more do they want from me?" However, she was regularly depressed by lack of phone calls or cards on holidays and then spoke of how hard it was to live with the guilt of knowing she had failed as a mother.

"I got a call from my oldest son last night. He's the only one who ever calls me anymore."

The sadness she felt was coupled with guilt. She wanted her children there for her, but simultaneously realized she had not always been there for them when they needed her.

"What positive memories do you have of your children?" This question elicits pleasant memories of when she was taking care of them.

"When they were all little, they would play, running around the house, getting into everything."

"Those are the precious moments that will always be with you, Connie, when you were taking care of them. Now it's time to take care of yourself."

Connie was followed in this way for about a year and a half before tragedy struck one of her best friends. This gentleman was a frequent guest and former lover. He, too, had been followed by the home care program for the last year. Andrew was admitted to the hospital and subsequently spent the last month of his life in a long-term care facility because of nonhealing cellulitis of both lower legs and uncontrolled diabetes mellitus. With the loss of her closest friend, Connie turned to the one stable individual in her support network, a seventy-four-year-old widower named George. George was now willing and able to provide Connie with a second home, transportation, and companionship. They had met about ten years before through mutual friends. Around his apartment were displayed photographs of Connie splendidly dressed, in better times. Although Connie's drug addiction puzzled and frustrated him, George enjoyed her company and was committed to helping her in any way he could.

When she moved into his apartment, she moved one step away from friends who were promoting her addiction to diazepam and heroin. Both Connie and George were counseled in biweekly visits. Having opposite lifestyles, they had difficulty adjusting to each other's demands. Connie's need to maintain her less-than-desirable friendships was supported by the home care team as long as she kept appointments and complied with her medication regime. George's demands, as caregiver, included smoking safety and decreasing diazepam use.

As months went by, Connie became accustomed to and surprisingly dependent on regular meals, showers, and medication. While the point was never reached where it could be said that Connie was no longer in danger of relapsing into substance use, the team's frustration was reduced by knowing she was in a safer environment, and that she was satisfied with her situation. By being a part of her safety net, the team helped her make choices that built her self-esteem. By accepting her as she was and consistently being both available and supportive, they helped her deal with past issues of failure. By supporting her chosen primary caregiver, they acknowledged and validated her desire for health maintenance.

Connie and George lived together for about eight months. She never again used heroin. They often would take a day trip to the shore or go out for a meal. She was able to enjoy visits with her grandson. They looked forward to a nurse coming several mornings a week to assess her worsening cardiopulmonary status secondary to her history of Cardio myopathy and baceterial endocarditis. She died suddenly in the hospital from an embolism, just minutes after a telephone conversation with George.

LESSON 14: ACCEPTING LIMITATIONS

In cases such as Connie's, the medical social worker is an invaluable resource for all drug-related issues. The social worker's experience and expertise provide the team with the information needed to cope with the lifestyle differences encountered in this population. It is important to be available for the active substance user even if it means waiting at the bottom of the cliff, prepared to pick up the pieces fall after fall. The medical social worker's care plan includes relapse prevention. This means anticipating the events that trigger a relapse: depression, loneliness, hunger, and pain. People can be given the tools to help themselves build a support network in the community. Drop-in centers provide companionship and meals. Counseling groups deal with depression, which becomes a particular concern at holiday time. Volunteers can provide transportation and companionship. The local chapter of AIDS education and resources may offer classes in various aspects of home maintenance and self-help as well as access to basic needs such as furniture and clothing.

Flexibility is essential to set goals with a person who appears to be living on a magic, flying carpet. In Connie's situation, goals were met by keeping expectations small. Short-term goals were symptom management, early intervention in symptoms of opportunistic infection, and relapse prevention. Realistic health-promoting behaviors in the areas of nutrition, hygiene, and appointment keeping were taught. In turn, unconditional acceptance gave her the confidence to trust her own judgment even if it meant occasionally making mistakes.

Methadone dispensation is regulated by the U.S. Food and Drug Administration. The guidelines specify frequency of dosing, frequency of clinic visits, and provision of counseling. Methadone can only be routinely prescribed by a physician for analgesia as Dolophine. It is illegal to prescribe methadone for chemical dependency outside of a federally regulated program. Methadone is a slow-acting, synthetic drug with properties similar to morphine. Methadone is the only effective treatment for heroin addiction. The dose is determined by the amount of heroin the individual used in the past and on subjective response and objective assessment by the clinical staff. The higher the dose, the more stored in the liver, available for time-release action. The effects of the drug are noticed after about thirty minutes and begin to wear off after eighteen hours. Its therapeutic effect lasts up to thirty hours. Each person receives a computerized measured dose of liquid methadone and is required to drink it under supervision.

Methadone is an effective drug for heroin users because it not only prevents withdrawal symptoms, but decreases drug craving. In addition, methadone blocks the euphoric effect of any other opiates (Woods, 1995). Methadone programs require random urine testing for drug screening to encourage compliance with program rules. In addition to one-on-one counseling, group counseling and support sessions are available for individuals or families, geared toward a variety of special interests.

Accepting responsibility for a patient's care needs to begin and end on a professional level. The goal is to enable the patients to help themselves and remain independent for as long as possible. It is important for home health care workers to recognize when their motives may be to make *themselves* feel needed or useful.

By frequent visits and phone calls, the message is sent that the individual is important. By following up on each clinic visit, reviewing changes, monitoring the effects of new treatments, assessing tolerance of new medications, and reviewing laboratory results, each individual's health status can be determined. By rescheduling missed appointments, ordering medication refills on time, and continually reassessing for new symptoms of opportunistic infections, individuals are encouraged to do the same.

There are no expectations of behavior. Success is measured in daily or weekly accomplishments. Success is taking advantage of each and every opportunity to educate. Success is accepting failure today and looking toward tomorrow as a new beginning. If we, as health care workers, are able to let go of personal responsibility for unmet expectations, the patient is also given permission to move on, start again, to begin counting the days of being drug-free once again.

Chapter 15

Beyond Belief

Paul was referred for home care follow-up by his father. Mr. Doe had heard about the program from his priest. He knew that Paul had AIDS and recognized that his illness was entering the terminal stages. In addition, Mr. Doe believed that Paul was actively using illegal drugs as well as abusing his prescribed drugs. He also believed Paul to be a danger to his wife and their two young children. Mr. Doe was desperately seeking help for Paul. Through the years, the repeated disappointments and heartaches that Paul's addiction had caused did not lessen his parents' love. However, they felt powerless to intervene effectively.

After discussing Paul's case with his primary physician and obtaining nursing orders for initial treatment, an appointment was made with Paul in his home. Often on admission, an active IDU is found to be homeless, hungry, uncomfortable, irritable, withdrawn, and living in an unsafe environment. Each of these areas is of equal importance and difficulty, but safety for the patient and household members is always the priority.

During the admission interview, Paul talked about his declining health, frustrations with his doctor, and recent thoughts of suicide. The admission nurse described him as "an agitated, angry, thin, thirty-four-year-old, living in a cluttered apartment." This description of his home was an understatement. Anyone entering would have been bewildered by the array of furniture and machinery filling the floor space of both rooms. In addition to the safety and fire hazard concerns, a family living arrangement seemed impossible.

Paul's somatic complaints were decreased appetite, irregular bowel activity, difficulty swallowing, and pain "all over, like arthritis." No bottles were available to confirm the medication prescriptions. Paul reported that he took Diflucan (fluconazole) daily, Mycobutin (rïfabutin) daily, Valium (diazepam) at bedtime, and Vicodin (hydrocodone) every six hours. He stated that he had been unable to speak to his present physician for several weeks and that he did not have an office appointment. Further, he said he believed that his present primary physician did not want to give him any more prescriptions for pain. Overall, he said, they did not have a good relationship. During the interview he spoke angrily both to and about his wife and about her lack of interest in his care. His wife, Sue, was ten years younger. They had been together for about four years and had a three-year-old son and a two-year-old daughter. Other than state assistance, he currently had no financial resources or employment history. He formerly had been working as an appliance repairman out of his own home. Sue was relying on family and friends to help with child care while she attended community college.

The following day, the social worker and primary nurse visited together to assess the need for psychosocial, medical, and psychiatric intervention. His CD4+ count was confirmed to be less than 50, putting him at high risk for opportunistic infections. On this second visit, Paul presented differently. Although still anxious, he no longer seemed angry. Both the social worker and the primary nurse were encouraged by his assurance that he intended to work with the team. It was explained that finding the right intervention might take a little time and that the goal was to decrease the stress in their lives and to address his physical discomfort. As the visit ended, he reemphasized that his most urgent need was pain medication.

The initial interventions for Paul were based on safety. He spoke of feeling suicidal. He was verbally abusive to his wife and children. His home was dangerously cluttered. He worked with electric appliances found in others' trash. The conditions existing in Paul's home were all addressed by the medical social worker through counseling and education over the next several months. A volunteer was found who shared Paul's interest in mechanics and was willing to spend some time with him. Privately, Sue was instructed in how and when to contact a shelter for women and children if she felt threatened by Paul's behavior.

His other obvious needs were pain management and nutrition. Paul described his pain as being "in my feet," and his gait reflected his discomfort. By improving telephone communication with his current physician, a short-term prescription for Vicodin was obtained. During this conversation, the best way to manage prescriptions in the future was discussed. It was mutually agreed that the team palliative care physician could better manage the pain medication through the reports of the team members based on frequent home visits. Over the following weeks, a progressive ladder of nonsteroidal anti-inflammatory drugs, short-acting and long-acting narcotics, and adjunctive medications was begun. After approximately three months, his prescription was upgraded to M S Contin (controlled-release morphine), with Vicodin for breakthrough pain.

Through the local AIDS chapter, Paul was able to obtain cases of canned nutritional supplements. Individuals are medically qualified for this benefit if they have a CD4+ count below 200, a diagnosis of AIDS, and have experienced a 10 percent weight loss. These supplements are a vital part of the nutritional program. Initially, Paul was provided with a case per week. He and his wife were given verbal and printed information on food purchasing, preparation, and economical recipes as well as the names of local food banks.

Paul was too physically debilitated to take a bus and could not afford to take a car or taxi to various appointments. Through the hospice volunteer department, Paul was eligible to receive transportation to medical appointments. Another available service is community-funded minibus transportation for medical appointments. While the door-to-door service of a volunteer is ideal, it sometimes creates another dependency. To foster independence, use of the minibus service is encouraged.

Ironically, as time went on and a trusting relationship was developed, Paul was forced to disclose that he was abusing and selling the medications the team physician was prescribing. The first indication of prescription abuse happened about a month after initiating the combination of M S Contin and Vicodin. At that time, Paul claimed that he had lost some of the tablets. The policy is that the patient is given the benefit of the doubt one time only. When he claimed that a car ran over his bottles of narcotics but spared the rest of his prescriptions, suspicions were aroused and he was confronted.

During one morning visit, Paul's primary nurse was unpleasantly surprised to watch him casually drop a handful of Vicodin into his coffee. The hospice physician immediately began limiting the amounts of pain medications to a weekly supply. At that point, the pain assessment focus changed to determine what might be the lowest effective dose range. Gradually, all pain medication was changed to nonprescription drugs, with little change in Paul's subjective response.

Paul was a classic example of how an IV drug user can excel at manipulating the system to obtain prescriptions for narcotics. He could mimic the actions and quote the symptoms of HIV/AIDS-related peripheral neuropathy. Paul's sincerity was questioned when he reported that the prescribed medications did not provide any relief for his symptoms and the nurse did not observe any change in behavior or functional level. The street value of prescription drugs is a necessary consideration when evaluating the reasons for poor response to a typical pain management regime.

Also during this time, the nutritional supplements were reevaluated. After several months of supposedly drinking three or four cans of supplement every day, Paul showed almost no weight gain. He repeatedly denied any gastrointestinal upset or diarrhea. In fact, his constipation persisted. When he requested case after case of supplements without visible signs of weight gain or change in bowel habits, their street value had to be considered. Again, the patient is initially given the benefit of the doubt, unless there is evidence to the contrary. In Paul's situation, proof was available; he was seen walking away from home with a case under his arm.

Paul began making excuses for missing clinic appointments. While the home care team acts as an agent of the physician for symptom management, any antiretroviral or prophylactic therapies need to be prescribed by the community physician. Therefore, in order to continue any aggressive or palliative care, office or clinic visits are vital. Not following through with appointments for medical evaluation reflected a lack of commitment to the plan of treatment. Home health care agencies operate according to physician's orders. When a patient refuses to be seen by a physician, it leaves the agency with no license to treat.

It is hard to write about Paul because a relationship based on trust and honesty was never established with him. He continued actively seeking drugs, haunting emergency rooms for pain medication, and missing appointments. When his wife left him, he lived alone for a few short weeks. From there he moved to a shelter for the homeless, until there was a bed available in a group home for PLWA. He was in the group home for less than two months, however, before his behavior became disruptive and abusive, and he was asked to leave. He moved back into the shelter, and resumed life on the streets. Within a few weeks, he befriended and moved in with another young woman. While a sincere attempt was made to keep in contact with Paul, the lack of a telephone or permanent address made connection impossible. Even more difficult was Paul's unwillingness to continue to work with a home health care team. Although efforts were never stopped, these obstacles to regular contact were never overcome.

This case sadly illustrates many of the problems encountered with care of IV drug users who are not ready to take the steps necessary to help themselves. Paul's addiction was the ultimate motivating factor in his daily life. For this he sacrificed family, friends, and his own health. While Paul's advanced disease and AIDS dementia played a part in his lifestyle choices, drug addiction ruled his life and caused his death.

Paul's wife and children were able to find support from her family, and remain together in their own apartment. Sue has continued with her plans to earn a college degree.

Paul's parents were followed closely by the team's bereavement counselor after his death. They were also referred to a bereavement support group for families of people with AIDS. Through grief counseling and support, they have been able to give themselves credit for changing all that they could change and to forgive Paul for being unable to change himself.

LESSON 15: SAFETY FIRST

Providing holistic care includes evaluating the safety of the patient's environment. An interdisciplinary team of home health care workers depends on documentation of events and evaluations by each member. The safety of the patient's family and community must also be taken into consideration. With the AIDS/IDU the plan for medication monitoring and management is integral. When evaluating the outcome of particular case, what is reviewed is whether standards were followed and interventions were appropriate.

After spending five or six hours racing between homes and clinics comes the time for the least favorite task: documenting the day's activities. While this is tedious, it is also critical for future reference. Other health care workers will need to rely on your documentation of phone calls, referrals, and interventions. Patients may also use this as a part of their medical or social history. Most important, the team will need to know what has been planned, how decisions have been made, who has spoken to whom, and the expected outcome.

How family members interact from day to day may vary. Anger in the household is heightened by the stress of disease. Providing support to each member begins with an assessment of interpersonal relationships. If there is potential for violence, the social worker needs to immediately provide information on community resources available for both emergencies and long-term follow-up.

To maintain consistency, prescriptions should be ordered from the same physician and pharmacy. If multiple caregivers are involved, one should be designated to coordinate the prescription pickup and administration of medication. If the patient is responsible for his own medication administration, it needs to be clear among all team members that medications will be refilled only at the prescribed time unless there are changes in symptoms requiring reevaluation of the prescription. This should be documented and communicated to the team regularly.

A health care worker brings a knowledge base to the job. Understanding what the agency expects from the employees is vital for workers to understand their jobs. Professional standards exist for all disciplines. Professional responsibility to the patient, the team, and the agency needs to be clearly defined. It is the responsibility of each professional to be aware of these standards and be willing to apply them to the challenge of caring for the AIDS/IDU.

Chapter 16

Running on Empty

Mark's story is one of inordinate human strength and endurance. His powerful will to survive on his own terms left his family with the gift of knowing he had persisted for the sake of attaining his own goals. He had learned this lesson from his mother, who was well acquainted with grief and hardship. Through it all, she taught her children the value of education and hard work. As she once again, at the age of fifty-nine, stepped into the role of mother to her three-year-old and five-year-old granddaughters, she also took charge of the care of her oldest son as he was dying of AIDS.

The referral for Mark's case came simultaneously with the referral to a home infusion company for intravenous hydration. He had not been able to eat or drink for four days. Mark had gone to the clinic the previous week, where he was told to "get his affairs in order" since he had a very short time to live. His CD4+ count had been between 6 and 10 for a year. He had survived PCP but had suffered uncontrolled weight loss for several months. The hydration was to be reviewed on a daily basis, since it was believed he would not survive more than a day or two. Over the next two weeks it became clear that, although he was not going to regain his strength or the ability to swallow easily, he was not ready to leave this world. He did not require encouragement to meet his own basic needs. As his own taskmaster, he was soon exercising, sipping, sucking hard candies, and crushing his own pills to regain some of what he he had lost. He had business to finish.

Their neighborhood was designated as one requiring an escort service for home health care workers. Their property, however, was strikingly neat. Several huge trees and a sandy play area took up most of the yard. In the remainder was the vegetable garden. It was in this garden that Mark had patiently and fastidiously worked over the previous weeks, despite the fact that he had increasing difficulty swallowing even liquids. He had required a cane to stand for the past month. A wooden chair was next to the garden's edge because he frequently took time out to catch his breath. In June, after all the plants were in, Mark found he could no longer climb the stairs to his room. His mother, who had taken the family into her home as Mark's health declined, exchanged bedrooms with her son. This allowed him to be on the first floor, curtained off from the living area, with easy access to the bath.

At the age of forty, Mark had come full circle in terms of his intravenous drug use problem. His involvement with alcohol and marijuana in high school had not prevented him from graduating and working to support a wife and baby by age twenty. After his marriage broke up, Mark renewed associations with friends who were involved with heroin. He alternately worked and hustled to support his new habit until he entered a drug detoxification program. It was here that he met the mother of his two young daughters. Mark succeeded in detoxification, but his new significant other did not. They maintained a stormy but consistent relationship over the next four years. At that time she received a two-year prison sentence for drug dealing. Mark knew his health was failing. He applied for disability and took over the full-time care of his daughters.

Mark was suffering from profound neuromuscular pain, which often accompanies wasting syndrome. For this he was started on Duragesic (a fentanyl) 25 mcg t/d patch every seventy-two hours, with morphine suppositories every four hours as needed. He was unable to open his mouth more than a few centimeters because of dental abscesses and thrush which occluded his palate. After a day of IV hydration, he was able to rinse his own mouth but could not swish effectively with nystatin, Xylocaine (lidocaine), or other solutions. The next trial was EMLA cream, a topical anesthetic (Nykanen et al., 1991). By painstakingly applying it first with a cotton swab and then with his gloved finger, he could progressively numb enough area to clean and clear small portions of his mouth. A month before, his teeth and gums had been so decayed that the dentist advised him to have general anesthesia for proper repair. However, after several weeks of this self-debridment with the EMLA cream, he was able to have the complete dental examination, but he declined further dental intervention. He continued to swish and swallow both nystatin and Xylocaine solutions, took oral antibiotics (twice a day) and antifungal medication (daily) for as long as he could swallow tablets.

Mark had MAI infection and rectal herpes. These infections were under control. He knew he had to take seven pills a day: Mycobutin (rifabutin) twice a day, and acyclovir five times a day. He needed Bactrim (TMP/SMX) for PCP prophylaxis, Cipro (ciprofloxacin) for dental abscesses, and Zithromax (azithromycin) for treatment of a recent bacterial pneumonia. This meant four more pills per day. In addition, he managed to take a multivitamin and was switched to oral medication for breakthrough pain, Percocet (oxycodone), one to two every four hours as needed.

Mark also needed nutrition. Because of neurological damage to his larynx, he had lost both his gag reflex and vocal cord function. His voice was reduced to a whisper. He was certainly hungry, however, and was determined to satisfy his body's cravings. He gained strength, but not much weight, on a diet of custards, oatmeal, and eggs. He was too proud to be fed, but would allow others to prepare his meals. He preferred to eat alone because the process was slowed by continual coughing and choking. Ironically, as his hydration state normalized, he developed diarrhea and increased pulmonary secretions. At this time scopalamine transdermal patches were available. Changing them every other day was effective at reducing both.

No sooner would a care plan goal be set for Mark than he would exceed it. His daily question was, "What needs doing today?" He soon had his home health aide driving him first to the clinic and then to the bank. Limits had to be set on errands and activities in which the home health aide could participate. After another week, he was independent and back to gardening.

At that point, it was his mother who needed support to cope with the changes in their lives. There were legal matters to put in order for custody of the children. Mark was already connected to a case management agency. He had a very clear idea of what he wanted for his daughters, but had been unsuccessful in obtaining a lawyer to draw up a legal document. The medical social worker was able to help him make these arrangements, which named his mother as legal guardian of both girls. In addition, Mark's mother also needed to finalize her own retirement plans and adjust to the loss of a third child.

Yet, Mark needed close medical follow-up. He was willing to attend monthly clinic appointments despite the difficulty of transportation, long waiting lines, and his poor prognosis. His CD4+ count had been less than 10 for three years. He had rampant opportunistic infections, wasting, and profound anemia. Despite it all, his smile could light up a room. He was offered but refused intravenous nutrition because an external catheter or subcutaneous port would alter his self-image.

During one of his last times in clinic, the nurse practitioner who had worked very closely with him over the years said, "Mark, you are dying!" Mark looked her in the eye and said in his whisper, "Yeah, right!" His physician wondered if he had some degree of dementia because of his repeated denial of his prognosis. However, Mark's actions demonstrated that he did know as he prepared. During the next three months, Mark saw his daughters into the fall, into day care and new schools, and into new warm coats and shoes to deal with the New England winter. He ate the harvest from his garden and he continued to plan for his family's future.

Mark's story is one of survival rather than a changed outlook on life. However, he and his mother needed the community support, skilled nursing, social service intervention, and home health aide assistance to enable him to be at home. He dealt with his problems by addressing them with the help of the appropriate team member who was readily available to encourage him. He gave his family the ability to accept his loss by his own courageous acceptance. He died suddenly at home. He had been seen by the nurse that morning and his sister brought him a meal in the late afternoon. His mother found him unconscious and breathing irregularly when she arrived home in the early evening. He died knowing his children were cared for and that they would remember him for his successes rather than his shortcomings.

LESSON 16: PROMOTING PHYSICAL COMFORT

The goals of traditional hospice care are centered around physical and emotional comfort. Once the medical diagnosis is confirmed, the short-term goals are education and pain and symptom management, while long-term goals center around promotion of comfort and a peaceful death at home. These are not the goals of the general health care system. Traditional medical care aims toward cure and treatment. In the home health care of PLWA, both short- and long-term goals are a variation on these themes.

To be effective, home health care agencies need both home care and hospice certifications to be able to offer the patient options in services. Through the home care model, active treatment in the form of antiretrovirals and protease inhibitors, intravenous medication or nutrition, and diagnostic medicine are all continued through the primary physician or clinic and are covered directly through primary insurance. Since AIDS has become a chronic disease, it is these treatments that maintain a person's functional level. The short-term goals for the dually diagnosed AIDS/IDU are home safety, meeting caloric and nutritional needs, education of patient and family, and compliance with the treatment plan. Long-term goals are early intervention in opportunistic infections and optimal functioning in the community. With disease progression, the patient needs to look at the option of palliative care. Although the short-term goals may remain the same, the long-term goals change to the traditional hospice model of comfort and a peaceful death at home.

Physical needs are immediate. An accurate physical assessment is necessary to sort out respiratory, cardiovascular, gastrointestinal, and genitourinary function. This is done on the first visit and thereafter at least weekly. Through a detailed pain assessment, the nurse advocates for the patient by relaying information to the physician, obtaining appropriate prescriptions, and assessing the effects of changes. When these needs are effectively dealt with, the psychosocial issues can be addressed.

With relief from physical suffering comes improved function. Also, the patient regains a sense of control over the situation. This often results in an improvement in attitude and situational depression, which in turn allows the nurse an opportunity to assess other aspects of the patient's physical and mental health. True symptoms of disease progression can now be assessed. An accurate evaluation of medication tolerance and compliance is necessary for effective treatment of bothersome or debilitating symptoms.

Social services, physical and occupational therapy, or nutritional counseling may be needed. Spiritual counseling is often welcomed by both the patient and the caregiver. It is most appropriate for a hospice home health care agency to enfold the dually diagnosed AIDS/IDU population because of the rainbow of nursing, psychosocial, and spiritual services they are able to provide.

Chapter 17

What If They Gave a Funeral
and Nobody Came?

Jill was diagnosed with AIDS several years before being referred for hospice care. On admission she reported her CD4+ count to be 10. She presented this information in a flat monotone. At 5'8" and 110 pounds, she was at high risk of being nutritionally compromised and recently began IV nutrition. The most recent addition to her medication list was Biaxin (clarithromycin) as prophylaxis for MAC (mycobacterium avium complex), which was causing diarrhea. She had been hospitalized repeatedly for bacterial pneumonia. She had learned to manage the self-infusion of TPN (total parenteral nutrition) as well as the care of a Hickman catheter. In addition, she was receiving prophylaxis for PCP, candidiasis, and recurrent genital herpes. A nurse from the home infusion company had been making home visits twice a week to administer intravenous Neupogen (granulocyte colony stimulated factor [G-CSF]) and to draw blood.

Jill's demeanor was as cold and impenetrable as marble. The brief eye contact she allowed did not reveal any insight into her inner state of mind. Jill made it clear that she did not want any changes in the people involved in her care. She was not happy with the idea of new people coming into her home.

A round of telephone conferences between Jill's primary care clinic and home infusion company resulted in the decision that the hospice home care would be the most appropriate single source of nursing to meet Jill's complex needs. Jill was introduced to the home care program gradually, slowly building trust by alternating home visits by individuals familiar to her with visits from the hospice home care nurse.

Jill, at age thirty-two, was used to being alone and independent. Even though she had been getting high with friends since her late teens, she had managed to support herself and her daughter. It was only in the past three years that she needed welfare and medical assistance to maintain her small neat home and her precarious health. She had worked intermittently as a waitress and in private clubs. Jill was unable to recall very much of what actually happened during these years. There were two risk factors in Jill's history: injection drug use and sexual contact with injection drug users. Currently she was maintaining a facade of functioning within her own home. Her rapidly diminishing energy levels and increasing memory loss resulted in overlooked meals, forgotten doses of medication, and compromised care of her daughter. In her favor, however, she was actively involved with Alcoholics Anonymous and in contact with a sponsor, which greatly reduced her risk for relapse into substance use. Of greater concern to her health care workers at that point was enabling her to deal with the internalized memories and the guilt that were consequences of those years of substance use.

Jill's twelve-year-old daughter, Renee, had recently been referred to a local mental health agency for counseling at the suggestion of her school counselor, based on recent changes in her behavior and academic performance. Because Jill was deeply concerned for Renee's welfare, she agreed with this intervention. How she actually felt about Renee being evaluated and having her own life indirectly examined was not something she was willing to disclose. Neither did she reveal any indication of guilt or remorse that she may have internalized.

Since Jill was involved with a case management agency for HIV-positive individuals and families, it was important to coordinate services with them. Through a joint home visit, the social worker and case manager coordinated a referral to a local mental health agency. The purpose of the referral was to counsel the daughter and Jill individually and together to help them deal with past unresolved conflicts and to provide a future resource for counseling for the daughter should anything happen to Jill. While recognizing the sensitivity of this issue, it had to be dealt with immediately due to Jill's failing health. Therefore it was presented openly and honestly to Jill, who gracefully accepted the offer of support.

After several weeks, Jill adjusted to the idea of new faces. She agreed to use a pillpack to remind her of the medication schedule, thus decreasing her risk for new or recurrent opportunistic infections. Being in her kitchen allowed regular assessment of her ability to shop, cook, and eat. Through meal planning and supplements, she gained some weight and avoided dehydration. When she reported having diarrhea, it was possible to quickly address its potential cause.

Although she had initially been well taught in the care and administration of fluids and medication through the Hickman catheter, she had lapsed into habits of poor technique and shortcuts which increased her potential for infection through the central line. She allowed the nurse to coordinate home visits to change the dressing and administer the Cytovene (ganciclovir) twice a week. By closely monitoring her laboratory work, her need for blood transfusions could be anticipated. Her risk of recurrent pneumonia was reduced by instruction and encouragement to follow prescribed inhaler and antibiotic regimes for upper respiratory infections and bronchitis.

One other major concern was her depression. The second was long-term custody and care of Renee. Both of these issues were dealt with primarily by the social worker in collaboration with the case management agency. Because Jill's mental state seemed to hinge on her ability to manage her own life and care for her dependent daughter, this was addressed gently. Through her primary care clinic, she was referred to a psychiatrist and prescribed an antidepressant. While her moods and affect remained flat, over the next month her functional status improved and she expressed satisfaction with her daily routine.

Jill only needed to be asked once if she had any spiritual concerns. Her surprised and open response was, "Well, of course I do. What do you think?" She had been considering calling her local parish for information about a home visit. After the initial phone call and introduction were made, she was able to follow through with future appointments. Her concerns centered around the religious education she had received as a child and her standing in the eyes of the church. The fact that a priest would visit relieved her mind.

Within a few weeks of overcoming this hurdle, Jill completed a durable power of attorney and a legal power of attorney for custody of her daughter, as well as discussing her general wishes for funeral arrangements. Any of these tasks is monumentally difficult for such a young person. The fact that she had the resolve and ambition to complete all three indicated her genuine desire to do the right thing.

Despite the stability Jill's case seemed to have reached, there remained a mysterious, stonelike quality about her. She answered any and all questions about her health and quietly cooperated with her schedule of appointments. She did not seem to socialize. She spoke occasionally about her brothers and sisters and their visits to her on weekends. Although she never said anything unkind about them, she did imply that they were of little help or support to her despite the fact that they all lived in the neighborhood.

Nursing visits continued twice a week as did monthly social work visits. In addition to the physical, psychosocial, and home safety assessments, she was observed for some indication of why she never let down her defenses.

One day she called the office to ask when the nurse was coming. Because of her severely impaired short-term memory, she had all her visits and appointments, as well as transportation arrangements, listed on a large calendar in her kitchen. When reminded of this, she replied that she needed to talk. The nurse was able to rearrange her schedule and go later that day, afraid Jill might forget what it was she wanted to say.

When the nurse arrived, Jill said, "You never asked me how I got HIV."

The nurse replied, "To me, Jill, it doesn't matter. It is more important to try to help you deal with the problems at hand. It is important to know an individual's risk factor for exposure to HIV for the purpose of anticipating risky behaviors that may result in new or recurrent opportunistic infections or health problems." The fact that Jill admitted to IDU had been documented as a primary risk factor.

"I have been thinking about those days lately. I just want you to know it wasn't my fault."

She was told, "I have a great deal of respect for you as a person, as a woman, as a mother, and for the way you are able to manage your life now."

"I don't know how it happened. I only remember that I went to this party with a guy I had been dating. That was when everything changed. Later, people told me that my boyfriend let his friends do whatever they wanted to me. I think that was the night I became pregnant, so I don't know who my daughter's father is. I think that's how I got the virus, too."

"You must think about that night a lot."

"I think that he betrayed me, but that I must have deserved it."

"No one deserves to be betrayed or to get HIV."

"For a few years I just didn't take care of myself or Renee. But then I cleaned myself up. I have tried. It has been very hard and I want people to give me credit for doing it. But all people do is criticize me for not doing more!"

"What made you think about this today?"

"I know I am getting sicker. I'm worried about Renee and what will happen to her. I want her to know that I really tried. I want my family to give me credit for what I have done right, not just blame me for the things I have done wrong."

"You're thinking about how people will remember you?"

"Yes, and I want to be remembered for some good things. I used to have a lot of friends. I only have my neighbor and my sisters and brothers now."

With encouragement, Jill brought all these issues to the psychiatrist she had seen in once before. She received professional guidance as well as continued encouragement from her home health team. She was visited regularly by the hospice team chaplain. Over the next few weeks she began to express her feelings about her siblings more openly. In turn, her family became more responsive to her needs for help at home and with Renee. Eventually, Jill was able to express her feelings about her past disappointments and regrets to her siblings. She was able to honestly talk about her addiction as well as her recovery.

Jill's internalized emotions were initially expressed as anger. She told her siblings that she resented their lack of faith in her ability to overcome her addiction and maintain her recovery. This, however, allowed her to express other positive emotions as well as her desire for forgiveness for past events. Jill allowed her inner beauty to be sculpted from the rock-hard, protective exterior she had built up around herself.

Jill recognized that her foothold of control was slipping. She agreed to a home health aide to assist with housekeeping and errands for two hours, three times a week. After maximizing state assistance services, these hours were then increased as needed over the following weeks through funding from community-based organizations in order to ensure her safety while family members worked during the day. As the important people in Jill's life spent more time with her, they learned more about AIDS and the difference between the myths of disease transmission and necessary precautions. Family members began to alternate evenings and nights so that Jill and Renee would not be alone.

The hospice nurse planned visits around times when a family member could be present to improve communication about the treatments she was receiving and to allow time for questions about what to expect in the future. The coordination of information among multiple family members fell on the shoulders of the home health team. When all team members including the home health aide were informed of Jill's options, there were fewer misunderstandings. As Jill's memory continued to worsen, a loose-leaf notebook was kept in the house to communicate among all the health care workers and family members. By recording recommendations, medications taken, vital signs, intake and output, and changes in condition, there was less chance of error or miscommunication.

By listening to what Jill was not saying, the home health care team identified potential gaps in family communication. By anticipating her needs, and by slowing down and stepping back from the situation, the team could objectively assess the response to the interventions.

If an individual's life can be judged by the number of people attending the memorial service, Jill's life was indeed a success. Her last wish was fulfilled as the church filled with people, gathered to remember her short life, as a tribute to her ability to overcome her addiction.

LESSON 17: ENSURING AND ENABLING PEACE

Recognition of the change from the chronic to the terminal phase of AIDS is easier from a distance. While onset of a virulent opportunistic infection, newly abnormal laboratory results, or a change in behavior may make this turning point obvious, it is more often a gradual process. When seeing a person on a weekly or biweekly basis these gradual changes often go unnoticed. Instead, weight loss, increase in fatigue, or memory impairment may be picked up in clinic. While this change in health status may not affect the daily routine, it may mean a revision of goals and care plan. What is important is that the change be recognized and communicated to all involved. Time is a luxury most AIDS patients do not have.

A person is entitled to the opportunity to face his or her own mortality. He or she may need to verbalize past experiences or frustrations and sort out current interpersonal relationships that are unbalanced.

There are several ways to work toward enabling peace of mind. The nurse should continue to address symptom management and promote communication between the patient and the primary physician. The social worker should coordinate psychosocial interventions. The home health aide should communicate daily changes in health status and home environment. If professional counseling or pastoral care is available, it should be offered, rather than assume that a patient's emotional or spiritual needs are being met. To overlook disease progression at any point is to deny the patient options for services. Provide each patient with the opportunity to find peace of mind.

Because of time limitations, only the present circumstances must be used as the starting point for changing behavior in the future. First and foremost is the acknowledgment that the past cannot be changed. Lack of self-esteem can prevent an individual from looking at the past objectively. Available choices in the present can be explored by accessing counseling either individually or through community support groups. Emotional and spiritual guidance is available through the hospice chaplain services at home. Also, patients need encouragement to utilize community spiritual counselors. By building self-esteem, accessing counseling, and encouraging the use of spiritual guidance, peace of mind can be achieved.

Chapter 18

Honor Their Journey

To remember José is to smile. His charm could light up a room and reassure the ones he loved that all would be well. He shared everything he owned and above all he was generous with his love. Although his Hispanic value system inhibited him from displaying his emotions, he eventually shared his fears in a quiet way.

José was twelve years old when he moved with his family from Puerto Rico, seeking relief from the high unemployment. They left behind their small house and farm near the ocean and followed other families to the large metropolitan area with affordable rent and access to factories which employed unskilled men and women. His parents planned to work hard and allow their children to take advantage of better educational opportunities.

José and his brothers and sisters found their dark complexions to be a disadvantage. In Puerto Rico they had affectionately called each other *negra* or *negrita*. They did not think of themselves as being part of the African-American culture. In fact, skin color had never been an issue.

The two oldest siblings, both boys, ages seventeen and eighteen, had the most difficult adjustment. They attended school, enduring the laughter at their heavily accented English and simple clothing. They missed the respect of their peers they had known in Puerto Rico. Although they quickly learned English, they were embarrassed to speak in class, thus drawing attention to themselves. The entire family felt that the coldness in this new city extended beyond the climate and temperature changes.

As a family they were united, maintaining their cultural identity, supporting and protecting each other. They did not make friends at school, but instead limited socializing to their Hispanic friends and neighbors.

All three brothers clearly understood their roles in the male-dominant, Hispanic family, following their father's example of using physical strength to gain respect within their neighborhood. Although they resented being ridiculed, they were not afraid of the other boys. Even if their father had not been heavy-handed in his discipline, they would have learned that machismo often required the use of force and aggression. Life in the city streets was a series of battles to be won at all costs. At age eighteen, José joined the army and served for four years. After his discharge, he returned home to find his older brothers making fast money selling drugs. José, too, developed an injection drug habit. The virus was transmitted through the needles they shared "getting high on the supply."

Over the next eight years, José's world was dismantled. His father had died soon after José returned home from overseas. When his two older brothers died from AIDS, José became the oldest surviving male. José had been motivated to stop injection drug use and participate in a methadone program several years before, but unfortunately he was already HIV positive. For the sake of his family he was determined to overcome his chemical dependency. By maintaining his recovery, he gained the respect of his family.

As a father figure, José would overcome his fatigue to instruct, reprimand, or feed his many nieces and nephews who frequented their apartment. He often performed home and automobile maintenance chores. In this way, despite his disability, he was able to fill the expected role of the family's oldest male. This was essential for José as a Hispanic man; it was also important to him because he felt he was deserting his family and thus failing to live up to their expectations.

Although he attended a clinic for regular medical follow-up, he had refused home care. When he came to hospice for palliative treatment of disabling symptoms, he was virtually homebound. His limited endurance restricted his activity to his own home or as far as a waiting car for the most necessary trips: monthly doctor's office visits and daily methadone clinic.

José had recently lost about twenty-five pounds. He was bothered by dyspnea on mild exertion, bilateral pedal and ankle edema, productive cough, sore throat, dry mouth, and dry skin. He was concerned about prominent varicosities across his abdomen and back and by abdominal swelling. He described burning in both feet and lower legs, abdominal cramping, and sharp, intermittent chest pains. The combination of these symptoms defined the advanced stage of his disease.

His medical diagnoses included MAI, oral candidiasis, peripheral neuropathy, advanced hepatitis, and community-acquired pneumonia. His CD4+ count was less than 10. An education program was started with both José and his family to relieve his most annoying symptoms. For dry skin, he was to shower daily and apply petroleum jelly to his arms and legs while they were still wet. José initially thought this would be unpleasant. However, he found that the ointment rapidly soaked into his skin and within ten minutes, he felt quite normal. After several days the flaking and itching was much improved.

To control the peripheral edema, he wore elastic stockings measured to fit his enlarged ankles and elevated his legs whenever he was sitting down. Although the edema never resolved, he was able to wear shoes and his gait stabilized.

José's medication list included treatment for the active infections and appropriate prophylaxis against other opportunistic infections. These totaled fifteen different prescriptions. Despite good intentions, he was unable to self-administer these accurately. He agreed to have the home care nurse fill a pillpack weekly to remind him of the dosing times. There are several advantages to this system. One is increased compliance with the prescription regime. A second is that missed prescriptions can be monitored to allow assessment of medication tolerance and side effects. A third advantage is that the need for refills or new prescriptions can be anticipated. By regular dosing of antifungals (for thrush), antibiotics (for pneumonia), and tricyclic antidepressant (for peripheral neuropathy and mild insomnia), some of Josés most bothersome symptoms were decreased.

As a part of the pain management program, the hospice physician coordinated conversion of the daily dose of methadone to transdermal morphine (fentanyl) by calculating the dose of morphine to equal the current dose of methadone. This relieved him of the daily strenuous trip to the methadone clinic while continuing to address his need for pain medication and to control his narcotic dependency. To relieve the breakthrough pain in his legs and abdomen, he was given morphine elixir. These types of morphine are very effective. They also eliminate the need for additional pills that need to be swallowed or accounted for. Both patient and caregiver must share their commitment to the same goal of comfort and increased functional ability.

José did have one episode of street-drug use while on the morphine, but he was honest when confronted. He admitted that he did not trust that he would be believed if he asked for more medication, and was surprised to be given a stronger dose of transdermal morphine. This dose did control both the drug craving and the pain he had been experiencing. It was agreed that a weekly pain assessment was needed and that his morphine dose would be adjusted to meet his needs.

In addition to hepatitis José had obstructed hepatic circulation and failure. Although this was irreversible, the symptoms of constipation and nausea were treatable. Perhaps more important, he and his family were reassured that the varicosities were not dangerous and would not rupture.

José's favorite time of day was noon. His mother, with whom he shared the apartment, usually went to Mass every morning, stopping at the grocer or drugstore on the way home. She would often stop at the *botanica* for the prescribed herbs for her arthritis and for José's cough. On special occasions she often purchased incense and candles to use in prayer to her favorite saints. When she returned, he could count on good things happening in the kitchen. Because his mother spoke only Spanish, the conversation was always a lively mixture of both English and Spanish. This too helped pass the time of day among the many friends and family members who came by.

José was relieved when it was decided during the first week of admission that a professional interpreter would be necessary to communicate with his mother. Although he did not like explaining his illness to her, it was important to him that she understand his needs. He was also acutely embarrassed when his young nieces or nephews were called upon to discuss his situation.

Evenings brought on the temptation to enjoy his old habit of drinking beer. A glance into the wastebasket would reveal several empty cans. "I only had one!" he would insist. Hepatic failure causes alcohol to be metabolized at a much slower rate, and every can of beer is an assault on the hepatic system. Even though the goal is to remain nonjudgmental regarding any substance use, patients need to know that certain drugs (such as alcohol in the case of liver failure) may hasten their death.

José did not like nighttime when he was left alone with his thoughts. Unable to sleep he sometimes stared at the religious images hung by his bed and the photograph of himself in his army uniform that hung over his bureau. To José, nights meant lying awake, listening to his ears ringing from severe anemia and wasting, napping only to wake in a sweat, having to get up and change his T-shirt and pillowcase. Nights also meant quiet time for thoughts about his two brothers who had already died from AIDS.

José had been visited by the same nurse two or three times a week for several months before he mentioned his aversion to nighttime. He then went on to say, "I dreamed about my brother last night."

The nurse replied, "I'm listening if you'd like to talk about it."

"He told me not to worry."

"About what?"

"I felt like he was there, right there for me. I think he is waiting for me."

The nurse was aware of the Hispanic belief that communication with others who have died is desirable, and that these spirits can provide support to the living. She also was aware of how difficult it was for José to speak about this with her.

She responded, "Many times, people feel or sense others they loved who have died. It is not unusual. Do you remember anything else about your dream?"

"I think when I die I will be with my brothers again. I am not afraid, but I do not know what it will be like."

José respectfully looked away when he said, "I decided that I want to die in the hospital."

The nurse asked, "What does dying in the hospital mean to you?"

José quietly replied, "I don't want a lot of fuss here at home. When my brother died the ambulance came and there was a lot of crying and yelling."

Reassuringly, the nurse said, "You are making the decisions for which treatments you want to receive and which ones you don't.

Your sisters and mother all have agreed to accept those decisions. You can decide what is best for you."

Several minutes went by before he said, "I don't want to have any pain."

Knowing José regarded her as an authority, the nurse confidently replied "I promise you, José, you will have enough morphine so that you will not have pain. The doctor is aware of your situation and is prepared to prescribe the right dose."

There was again a significant pause before José admitted, "I am ashamed of some things I have done in the past. I know I have disappointed my family at times."

The nurse replied, "José, I have been coming to see you a lot for the past three months. I have spoken to your family many times. They have said over and over how much they love and respect you. They are willing to help you through this and are not going to leave you alone. They will always love you."

José was experiencing the normal fears of advancing AIDS: fear of pain, dependence, dementia, humiliation, and dying alone. At the same time he worried about the emotional impact his death would have on his family.

By acknowledging and validating these fears as normal, José was given permission to think further about some important contributions he had made to his family and his home. He regained his sense of control through effective, regular pain management and readily available prescriptions for nausea, sleep, and anxiety. Through family discussions with the nurse and the medical social worker, he was reassured that he would be remembered with honor.

LESSON 18: UNSUNG HEROES

Hispanic Americans are defined by the U.S. census bureau as people speaking Spanish or of Spanish, Portuguese, or Latin American descent. In 1990 there were 22,400,00 Hispanic Americans in the United States. This was an increase of 53 percent over the previous ten years. It was estimated then that this number would increase to 30 million by the year 2000, and to 40 million by the year 2010, bringing the number of Hispanic Americans to 13 percent of the total U.S. population, equaling the percentage of African Americans (Katz, 1993).

The majority of Hispanic Americans live in southern Florida, Texas, New Mexico, Arizona, Colorado, and California. However, over one million Hispanic Americans live in New York City, equaling one-quarter of its population. Nevada and Rhode Island have the fastest growing number of Hispanic families, followed by Virginia, New Hampshire, and Massachusetts (Katz, 1993).

Cultural sensitivity goes beyond race and ethnicity. It involves developing an awareness and appreciation of the values within a culture. These values define right and wrong, influencing the way an individual both thinks and behaves. Programs that are culturally sensitive are able to effectively address the specific cross-cultural situations of the minority populations they are trying to serve.

Ignoring culturally specific needs of the patient or family may result in blocking access to resources. This attitude does more than reflect a lack of manners; it is oppression that results in creating powerlessness for those involved to either influence or change their surroundings. Some strategies to remember are:

- Learn about the culture.
- Ask questions if you do not understand.
- Learn the family members' names and relationship to the patient.
- Do not use a child as an interpreter.
- Respect the fact that you are a foreigner to this family.
- Anticipate that past experience with insensitive programs and people may have caused suspicion and resentment.
- Include all family members in the patient's care.

Culture often determines attitudes about self-care practices and health care. These attitudes have physical and psychological effects on the outcome of medical therapies, influencing the patient and family to accept or reject prescriptions, treatments, and advice. Members of the first generation to a community bring with them a full set of values regarding how to prevent and treat illness. These beliefs are based on their own personal experiences as well as those of generations past for accepted, traditional management of illness. Subsequent generations are more likely to be receptive to scientifically based medical practices. It is not uncommon for ethnic patients to seek help simultaneously from both a folk healer for traditional remedies and a physician for a prescribed treatment.

By understanding the meaning and importance of traditional beliefs and treatments, the health care provider can work toward integrating scientific practice into a plan of care.

Puerto Ricans in New York City seek help for their health problems from a variety of sources, such as neighborhood herb shops (botanicas) and doctors, but chronic or "spiritual" illnesses sent them to seek the aid of a spiritualist. In either individual or group seances, the spirit medium must locate the spiritual agent causing the illness and identify the spiritual strengths of the patient. Once the cause has been found, one or a combination of treatments must be carried out to remove the negative spiritual influence, usually through exorcism, "working the cause" (convincing the spirit to leave the person alone), or prayer and ritual, sometimes accompanied by herb or medical treatment. (Thernstrom, Orlov, and Handlin, 1980, p. 458)

Within the Hispanic culture, "the family is regarded as the hearth, the sustaining warmth. It is almost a political party, the parliament of the social microcosm, the security net in times of trouble. And when have times not been troubled?" (Katz, 1993, p. 17). Family loyalty has been undermined in mainland America by the pressure to be successful and obtain an education. As with other immigrant groups in the past, the conflict between first and second generations further weakens the traditional relationships among extended family members. This can leave the current population of young Hispanics living with AIDS without the traditional support system.

A strong Hispanic tradition is the respect of authority figures, including all health care providers. It is considered disrespectful to disagree with someone in a position of authority. Overt disagreement would be considered rude, making the authority figure uncomfortable. Lack of eye contact implies respect rather than defiance or avoidance. This philosophy extends to the respect of children for their parents. The patient may be embarrassed if intimate issues are discussed either in front of a child or by using him or her as an interpreter.

Machismo is a code of behavior exclusive to Hispanic men. In order to be macho, men are expected to behave fearlessly, using physical power and aggression as necessary to maintain dominance. The aggression and bravado that fuel this behavior are similar to emotions felt by soldiers at war. Persistent street violence within metropolitan areas supports this competition for survival. Expressing emotions such as sadness or remorse reveals vulnerability and weakness, inviting rejection and loss of respect.

In the terminal phase of AIDS, it can be anticipated that fears will be concrete and focus on immediate changes: physical suffering, pain, nausea, insomnia, weakness as well as fear of disfigurement, dependence, and dying alone. While these are justified, they may be unacceptable to the male machismo. Fears need to be openly addressed. When faced with death, people review their lives. They become introspective. One or two sentences will open the door to invite discussion. While some people may benefit from more elaboration, many simply need to hear the words. "It's okay to be afraid." "Your life has meaning." "You will not be alone." "You will not be in pain."

Within the machismo, male-dominated culture, men are entitled to respect from all women. This respect is based on the male's superior physical power. Although, in turn, women are entitled to loyalty and protection from men, this does not extend into the realm of sexual relationships. "In a traditional Puerto Rican family, the man makes the decision for the household, accepts responsibility for its support, and is granted much more freedom than the woman in the disposition of his life and sexual behavior" (Thernstrom, Orlov, and Handlin, 1980, p. 863). This attitude of dominance over women becomes problematic when teaching health promotion and safer sexual practices. Men are reluctant to take advice from a woman. Men are far less likely to respond to their partner's request to practice safer sex.

Bravery is described as defiance, valor, or courage. Machismo requires bravado. In the situation of the dually diagnosed AIDS/ IDU, the definition of bravery may center around the adversity that they have overcome. The simple act of coming home after living on the streets may require immense courage. The fact that addiction has led to a life of social marginalization may mean that new courage is needed to face family and friends who were once ignored. In the battle with AIDS, the opponent is invisible and furtive. The tactics include ambush and four-flank attack. The weapons are acute opportunistic infections, insidious fatigue, neuropathy, and dementia. Living with AIDS means learning how to recognize the enemy, which battles to fight hard, and when to make peace. Those who muster bravery for this final stage of living are truly our heroes.

Chapter 19

The Grand Canyon

Fred was referred to hospice by his counselor at the methadone clinic. He was described as physically and emotionally exhausted from complications of advanced AIDS. His counselor stated that he needed help accessing community resources for himself and his family as a direct result of his disability. In addition, Fred needed coordination of his medical care because he wanted to change physicians and clinics.

On admission to the home care program, Fred appeared physically and emotionally exhausted. He was emaciated and described appetite problems such as anorexia and early satiety. He explained that he wore a brace on his lower left leg due to a "war wound." The way he described his neuropathic pain in both legs and feet could have been quoted from a textbook. He reported that he had been treated both recently and in the past for pneumonia. He had a diffuse skin irritation often seen in endstage AIDS: dry, flaky, itchy skin on all extremities and throughout his scalp.

Psychosocially, Fred's concerns centered around his family and the methadone program. His wife and two small children were present during the admission. His wife, Margaret, said she had been tested for HIV and was negative. Therefore, we knew that their two children, ages five and seven, were also negative. Although it was not apparent on this initial visit, it soon became clear that Margaret, too, had problems with chemical and alcohol use. Fred was looking for daily transportation to the methadone program, but he particularly had a problem getting there on weekends. He said that, although he wanted to attend regularly, he found the daily trip overwhelming.

Fred had been receiving health care from a Veterans Administration outpatient clinic for the past few years. Recently, he had been given prescriptions for progressively increasing doses of Vicodin (hydrocodone) and Percocet (oxycodone). He claimed he was dissatisfied, however, with the care he had received at that clinic. He had gone to the emergency room of another major hospital and had been referred to the immunology clinic, and given an appointment with the nurse practitioner. At that time he was denied prescriptions for narcotics until he was examined by a physician. He did receive Zantac (ranitidine) and Bactrim (TMP/SMX). He was told he would have to return to the clinic the following week. In the meantime, some initial blood work was done. After confirming this information with the nurse practitioner in the clinic, the home care nurse and Fred agreed that this was the necessary course of action. Fred had a small supply of Percocet and Vicodin on hand. He agreed to limit his activities and use this supply only as needed. Fred was assured that the hospice team would advocate for him once he was connected to a primary physician.

Over the interim weekend, Fred called to say that he was out of Vicodin and Percocet. The nurse on call asked him about the supply of medications he had had two days before. He said that he had needed to take them. He was informed of our inability, as nurses, to write prescriptions, and was reminded of the agreement that he would need to see a primary physician in the clinic the following week for further narcotic prescriptions. It was suggested that he return to the emergency room at any time that he felt severe pain. Fred calmly informed the on-call nurse that he thought that the emergency room would not be necessary because he did have five 100-mg M S Contin (controlled-release morphine) tablets that a friend had given him. He thought he probably would be all right until next week. While the sharing of medication is not condoned, home care workers must acknowledge the reality that it is a common coping and/or survival mechanism on the streets.

Later that evening, his brother, Al, called and asked for information and advice. He had just left Fred's house. Fred had informed him of his HIV-positive status and that he was now actually dying of AIDS. Al was distraught. He talked and cried to the nurse on call for over an hour. He said he had been bringing Fred to methadone on weekends off and on for a year. Al said that Fred's drug problems dated back many years; he had always tried to be available to him when he was in trouble. He wanted to know how to help him now. He wanted to know what to expect next. Due to the need for confidentiality, the conversation centered around how hospice generally helped people with AIDS and the problems associated with it and other terminal illnesses. Al was reassured that Fred would receive expert medical and nursing care. He was told about palliative and hospice care and the availability of professional nursing support twenty-four hours a day.

Fred presented as a polite, congenial person. His mannerisms were gentle and his voice was soft. Although on most visits he seldom finished a sentence without nodding off, he always apologized for falling asleep. At 5'10" and a slight 110 pounds, he was significantly underweight. He was thirty-eight years old, fair-skinned, and wore his hair pulled straight back in a pony tail because he liked the "long hair look of the 1970s." He said his philosophy of problem management was to deal with each day as it came.

Similar to many of the hospice referrals, he and his family presented in crisis. The team responded quickly, and developed a plan of care to address each of this family's major problems. He was asking for symptom management, advocacy with connection to a medical clinic, and transportation to his methadone program. He and his wife had no means of financial support. His wife had recently lost her job and was unable to find another. Because she, too, appeared to have substance use issues, the health and safety of the children was of concern. Fred said he needed support because he had not been able to share his health problems with anyone other than his wife and his brother.

In response to the potential crisis involving the children, the social worker contacted a local family mental health support center. Margaret agreed to follow up on the appointments made for herself and each of the two children together and individually. With permission, it was a relief to receive confirmation that Margaret's HIV test had been negative eliminating concern regarding the HIV status of her children. Applications for Social Security benefits and food stamps were filed. A resource list of local self-help and support groups was compiled and reviewed in detail with both Fred and Margaret. The family was referred to a case management agency for home follow-up. Education on nutrition, food safety and preparation, safe sex, and home management was begun by the social worker and nurse. Relapse prevention counseling was coordinated with Fred's methadone counselor, the initial referral source.

Although transportation to the methadone program could not be provided, a volunteer took Fred to the Division of Motor Vehicles to get a bus pass. He was referred to the local AIDS chapter for nutrition supplements and support. His family was promised that "things would get better" and that their circumstances were not unique.

A pharmacy concern arose during the third week Fred was on the program. After seeing the nurse practitioner, Fred had been given new prescriptions. When he did not have his refills, and was complaining of gastric distress, the pharmacy was called and asked about the status of these prescriptions. Although Fred had listed one store as his preferred pharmacy on admission, he had not left the prescriptions to be filled in that store. When questioned, Fred said he did use two other pharmacies from time to time, and that he must have taken the prescriptions to one of them.

Because of the difficulty of managing multiple prescriptions in multiple stores, Fred was asked to choose one pharmacy. During this coordination it was learned that Fred had a complex arrangement for refilling a long list of medications. Individuals who receive medical assistance have prescriptions paid by the state. These prescriptions and their costs are tracked by a statewide computerized network. Because he had paid cash for many of these prescriptions, a problem had never been recognized in a computerized, state-regulated system. The nurse was able to help Fred obtain all these prescriptions and fill a pillpack to help regulate his medication.

When the long-awaited medical appointment arrived, the nurse met Fred in the clinic to advocate for symptom management by speaking directly to his physician. He was prescribed low dose, long-acting morphine and Vicodin for breakthrough pain. The physician was concerned that Fred was changing doctors and clinics at such an advanced stage in his disease. Following the clinic practice of retesting all new HIV-positive patients, Fred was given an appointment to return to clinic in two weeks for results.

Over the next few weeks, the nurse visited twice a week to do a physical assessment, patient and family education, fill his pillpack, and coordinate refills of medication as necessary. He was monitored for compliance with the medication regime and for symptoms of developing opportunistic infections. The social worker followed up on referrals and continued weekly psychosocial counseling and support.

The results of his blood work from his first clinic visit were a surprise. The nurse practitioner called to confirm that the results showed a CD4+ count of over 1,200. She agreed to repeat the test. Dealing with a population who struggled daily with the devastation of AIDS, we were reluctant to believe that any person or family could possibly benefit from this diagnosis. No family would endure the stigma of AIDS unnecessarily. How anyone could subject their extended family to the agony of a potentially life-threatening disease was difficult to understand.

When the new results were confirmed and Fred was confronted in clinic, his reaction was not unlike his reaction to other situations. He calmly denied that he could either be wrong or misinformed. His physician was somewhat surprised by Fred's lack of enthusiasm about the good news. He surmised that Fred had learned of the recently passed federal guideline that the diagnosis of drug addiction alone would not qualify an individual for benefits. Fred no longer qualified for the home care program. He did not have AIDS or any other life-threatening illness. He was referred back to his counselor at the methadone clinic and his family referred to the community mental health agency.

Fred called the office six months later to say that hospice had caused the revocation of his Social Security benefits. He politely asked if he could be reconsidered to confirm that he was indeed ill. Fred was informed that the home care agency did not decide anyone's health status, that it was entirely up to his physician to make that determination. Although the agency could assist in the application, it did not have a role in determining qualification for benefits. He was advised to speak to his physician about both his health and his qualification for benefits. Fred had survived by developing his ability to quietly manipulate others and the health care system. Managing his addiction had become his career.

LESSON 19: PITFALLS TO AVOID

When dealing with addictive behaviors remaining on firm ground means avoiding the pitfalls of success. They include entrenchment in the patient's personal problems, being judgmental, acting on assumptions, or lack of professional boundaries.

Although many of us have used verbal manipulation to fulfill a desire from time to time, the IV drug user may have transformed it into both an art and a science as a means of survival. Do not expect this to change. Declarations of intentions to end a relationship or change a behavior are only the beginning in a rehabilitation process. This is not because the patient does not want it to happen, but because the combination of psychological and physiological dependency is beyond control. What can be accomplished is to open up communication among all involved. The patient, the health care team, and the community support network need to consistently abide by one plan of care. A family meeting provides the opportunity for everyone involved to hear the same information. Realistic choices can be offered and the patient and others involved can accept or reject those choices. Also, each team member's role and duties is clear to all.

Professional boundaries should not be fuzzy. If an action is within a job description and can be accomplished within the normal work day, it is both appropriate and expected. If unsure, a health care worker can ask, "Why am I doing this?" The answer should always be because it is within the plan of care and the plan of treatment.

Choices are always available. The patient, as the responsible person, must be the one to make them. This applies equally to small decisions about daily activities or about dire situations. It is the health care worker's job to carefully assess the patient's ability to understand choices. Instruction should be given at the patient's level. Also, it is important to include information about consequences that may follow naturally as a result of certain choices. Future prospects for basic needs such as housing, income, and interpersonal relationships with friends or relatives should be made clear. To allow an individual the opportunity to make a choice is to (1) give away that responsibility, (2) empower that person rather than yourself, and (3) allow time and space for that person to benefit from the information given and its application to daily living.

Chapter 20

Refilling the Empty Vessel

The following stories come from seasoned nurses who have found career satisfaction and personal fulfillment as specialists in care of the individual dually diagnosed with IV drug use/AIDS:

The last time I saw Pamela as an outpatient was the afternoon I met her in the emergency room. Her primary physician was also there. She was as yellow as a canary, and even then, she never stopped talking. Her dementia was so bad, she could not remember my name. I had been seeing Pam two to three times a week in her home for the past year and a half. She had been staying clean for the past few months. She was afraid to be admitted to either the hospital or the hospice inpatient unit because she knew she might never go home again. Her doctor coaxed her by promising that he would be able to help her to be more comfortable, and that it would just be for a little while. Actually, the fact that she was so demented made me feel better. She couldn't remember her grief, and, therefore, was happy during this very sad time. She taught me look on the positive side of everything.

Ralph told the most outrageous stories. He was so far out of reality, it forced me to be grounded. My favorite story is about the Christmas Eve that his wife was hit by a laundry truck while crossing the street (he was never married). He said she was dragged for three blocks before the driver realized she was there. She did not survive, of course, leaving Ralph with either six or seven children to support. He also was full of stories about his eighteen brothers and sisters. His adoptive parents told us he had been an only child. He was especially proud of the fact that he was a businessman. He carried business cards with just his name in bold letters advertising himself as a "Security Man." The fact that there was neither a telephone nor address was fine since he was homeless most of his adult life. The first time he received a Social Security check, he decided to spend it on a weekend at the Holiday Inn, enjoying the jacuzzi. On Monday he returned to Traveler's Aid.

Warren made me laugh. He was just a delightful man. When he was up and about he would cook enough food for an army and eat most of it himself. His favorite sandwich was disgusting sardines. One night, when he could hardly get off the couch, he called 911 because he dropped the remote control for the TV. He explained to the paramedics that he had fallen, but had managed to get back onto the couch just before they arrived, and, since they were there, would they please hand him the channel selector?

I feel I make a difference. Most of my patients have no life. But they have the potential for being good people.

Working with the IDU is particularly satisfying. They come such a long way with a little respect and care. At first every one presents a hardness as a defense. This is like a tough facade. They can't let anyone help them. They are really afraid. But after a few weeks, it's not hard to get their attention and respect. It's amazing what a positive response you can get by just treating an IDU, people we have labeled as our burden on society, with respect. I find that if you give respect you get it back.

One day, my patient Jeff said to me, "I was talking to my friend, Al, about how much my nurse helps me with my illness. Al became really annoyed and loud and he said, "Oh no, *my* nurse is the best! She made me realize I am worth something!" So the two continued to bicker about whose nurse was the best until Al asked, "What's her name?" This is when they realized they were both talking about the same nurse. I felt flattered by their loyalty, but more than that, I felt proud that through my efforts they had come to value their health.

Living in a small community has disadvantages. One is the concern for maintaining confidentiality. There are also advantages. The IDU community is well linked and when one dies they all grieve. They are able to provide support for each other. My patients are always coming up to me and talking about their friends, their situations, not knowing that I know the same people. I feel like I am part of the community and that I have an impact on the community through education and harm reduction.

Sometimes I'll see a certain one of my patients with some buddies, acting rude and obnoxious, which is completely different than when we are together. At times like that I'd like to kill him! So the next time I see him I give him a lecture about manners; he always smiles and tells me not to worry about him.

Bambi was sent to prison after she stole her mother's television. At that time she had been using heroin and cocaine on a daily basis. She weighed about 100 pounds and most days she could hardly make it up the stairs to her apartment. She had recently recovered from acute endocarditis. I went by her house two to three times a week. Every single time I would do teaching about the negative effects of drugs, especially with the virus. Many days she would hardly be able to keep her eyes open during the visit.

I would say to her, "If you want to live, think about yourself and your family." Her children had been in foster care their whole lives, but Bambi kept in touch with them.

Even then, I could appreciate the kind of person Bambi was, though. She would always protect me. If there were people in her apartment, she would come downstairs and tell me not to come up. I wasn't afraid that they would hurt me, but they might have taken my bag or my watch to sell. I was grateful that she cared enough about me to do that.

Bambi is like a miracle. I know now that she really listened. Now she says to me, "You were right. Everything you said about drugs was right. All I used to care about was where to get the next hit." Bambi spent six months in prison. When she was released she moved directly into a group home. She weighs over 160 pounds. She has been invited to speak at community events. She only needs to go to clinic every three months.

Progress is made in the relationship when patients feel able to admit that they get high. I never asked Cindy if she was using drugs. She volunteered to tell me because she trusted me and trusted our relationship. With this information, I can help her doctor to sort out if she is having symptoms of disease progression, side effects of medication, or if it may be related to street drug use. Cindy once explained, "You look at me as a person period. Not as an IDU."

Although Manny and I did not hit it off right away, I have seen a radical change in him. He was withdrawn and avoided visits for several months. I had to start calling him early in the morning, waking him up, to catch him at home, telling him I was on my way to visit. Now, he calls to say, "I miss you." He is a big, tough guy with a heart like a teddy bear. I teach him about how to avoid opportunistic infections. I tell him about toxo, MAI, AIDS dermatitis, PCP, and herpes and the importance of having treatment early. He sits there and complains, "I know, I know." Manny's sister died from AIDS. He has seen a lot of the bad times. He doesn't like to be reminded of the fact that he has AIDS. I tell him now, though, that if he is not going to be home, to let me know. "Don't waste my time!" And that when he needs me, I'll be there for him.

Once, after a few days of doing drugs, Manny's viral load went way up. After being clean and taking his medication for two weeks I was able to say, "See how your viral load has gone down!" He began to listen. He said, "Thank you." To me that is the biggest reward.

You never know what is going on in a person's mind. There is no immediate feedback. You have to convince them that you care about what happens to them. This is easy when you really do care. They are each unique individuals living in a culture all their own. They are the underdogs.

Kim was a tough, hard junkie with some mean-looking friends. I was with her when they came by one day. I said to her, "They only come to get you high. You look so good today. Can you go to visit your mother?" She agreed. Kim was admitted to our program with a viral load of over a million. Her CD4+ count was fifteen. The plan was to monitor her at home while she visited the clinic for a prescription of Klonopin on a weekly basis. She had completely stopped all her other medication because she said it made her feel worse. After two months, she is allowed to go every other week. Her CD4+ count is 160 and her viral load is 17,000.

I love my job. It makes me feel like I make a difference. Just a smile. Just being handed an empty pill pack by someone who has been nonadherent, is my reward. I wake up every day and I thank God for my life, that I have food and a safe home.

Wilbur had spent his adult life in prison. He was known as a cold, tough character. He expressed neither regret nor apology for his lifestyle. He had shown little or no emotion during the eighteen months of home care visits. That's why his gratitude was apparent when he innocently asked, "Will you marry me?"

I'll always remember a remark that Billy made. I don't think his intention was to be profound, but his expression of gratitude included one of the ironies of the culture of IV drug users in America today. He said, "I have spent my whole life hating white people. Now, they are the ones taking care of me in my last days."

And, finally, from a person whose life has been an emotional desert, who has survived rejection, abuse, and isolation, "Bye, I love you."

LESSON 20: LESSONS WE HAVE LEARNED

As a home care team specializing in the care of people with AIDS, we have experienced the culture of this population. Although at the beginning we were all at varying stages of innocence about drug addiction and related behaviors, none of us can claim that now. The reality of human shortcomings is part of the daily routine. By developing a level of comfort with this population, we have developed a degree of expertise.

A question we are asked regularly is "How do you *do* this work?" In other words, how do team members deal with the devastating, depressing, and potentially dangerous each and every day? While it is a rhetorical question, the team has discussed this and has some enlightened answers. Simplistically, we have learned to focus: set short-term goals, celebrate small progress, and expect nothing in return. We are searching for the key to open the door to each person's release.

Our goals are based on the mission of the agency, which is to improve the individual's quality of life, promote safety, and ensure comfort. Long-term goals focus on maximizing functional abilities, pain and symptom management, and harm reduction for both the individual and the community. Short-term goals include early intervention with opportunistic infections, education of patients and caregivers about nutrition, medication, dementia, and communicable diseases, how to access community services, and to promote adherence to a plan of treatment. The health care worker is not a friend, but an advocate to encourage and enable safe, independent living.

In the end stages of AIDS, people may eat without absorbing, go through the day without remembering, take medications that worsen their discomfort and damage other body systems, and accept throbbing pain with each step taken. They may live with emotional pain that cannot be reduced by any medication, and often lack the mental acuity for proper decision making. These ironies are compounded by the issues of lifelong addiction. It requires a long and arduous journey to prove to themselves and their loved ones that their lives will have meaning. The only proof of rehabilitation may be death itself. The sacrifice required to prove sincere love for family and friends may be dying alone. Fears are often only quieted by numbness; the road to peace may be blocked by humiliation; laughter may be checked by tears of regret.

As disease progression occurs, priorities follow those of the patient and caregivers as they accept the inevitability of dying. The short-term goals become relief of physical, emotional, and spiritual discomfort and enhancing a peaceful environment.

Perhaps the single largest obstacle to successful intervention with this population is recognizing that it is impossible to help someone who does not want to be helped. It is important to recognize the point at which the health care team is working harder than the patient. The objective is to make an impact without making promises. Because the future is uncertain, one way to do this is to visit as often as necessary to build trust. Unlike agencies for rehabilitation (such as methadone maintenance, Alcoholics Anonymous, or Narcotics Anonymous), time is not on our side. We must reach out, make ourselves available, and recognize and deal with the urgent needs while simultaneously teaching self-help and building self-esteem. We support the patient's and caregiver's efforts knowing that it is up to them to find the turning point to caring about themselves.

To advocate for this population, nurses, social workers, case managers, and physicians must have knowledge, capability, and willingness. These are the three qualifications needed to be able to succeed at working with an HIV/AIDS/IDU population. To successfully do this type of work requires a combination of smarts and guts. If someone has the knowledge and the willingness, but lacks the determination required to set limits and recognize manipulative behaviors, that person will not succeed. Some people have the knowledge and the capability, but may quickly find that this is not the culture they want to be involved with. Capability and willingness are not enough to meet this population's complex needs unless there is the knowledge base or desire to learn about the diseases of HIV/AIDS and addiction. Without this knowledge base the practitioner may miss the primary problem or the subtle signs of an opportunistic infection, thus losing the benefit of early intervention.

After the initially overwhelming sense of injustice passes, the depth of the needs and the vastness of deprivation is energizing. The ability to make a difference within one life and for one community becomes a daily reality.

References

Introduction

Day, Dawn (1997). "The Spread of Drug-Related AIDS Among African Americans and Latinos." *Health Emergency,* a pamphlet. Special Report by the Dogwood Center, Princeton, New Jersey.

Department of Health and Human Services (1997). "Needle Exchange Programs in America: Review of Published Studies and Ongoing Research." Report to the Committee on Appropriations for the Department of Labor, Health and Human Services, Education and Related Agencies, Washington, DC.

Duncan, David (1995). "A New Direction for Drug Education Harm Reduction." *The Catalyst, 22*(2), a report by the New York State Federation of Professional Health Educators, pp. 8-9.

Duncan, David, Nickolson, Thomas, Clifford, Patrick, Hawkins, Wesley, and Petosa, Rick (1994). "Harm Reduction: An Emerging New Paradigm for Drug Education." *Journal of Drug Education, 24*(4), pp. 281-289.

Editorial (1998). "Needle Exchange Programmes in the USA: Time to Act Now." *The Lancet, 351,* p. 75.

Lurie, Peter and Drucker, Ernest (1997). "An Opportunity Lost: HIV Infections Associated with Lack of a National Needle Exchange Program in the USA." *The Lancet, 349,* pp. 604-608.

Lyons, Catherine (1996). "Harm Reduction in Practice: Applications in an HIV Clinic." Poster presentation at the ANAC Conference, Chicago, Illinois.

Rosenbaum, Marsha (1997). "Kids, Drugs, and Drug Education. A Harm Reduction Approach." Policy statement by the National Council on Crime and Delinquency, The Lindsmith Center, San Francisco, California.

Wartenberg, Alan and Samet, Jeffrey H. (1992). "The Drug-Using Patient." In Libman, Howard and Witzburg, Robert (eds.), *HIV Infection: A Clinical Manual,* Second edition. New York: Little, Brown & Co., Inc.

Chapter 1

Snyder, Carol, Kaempfer, Suzanne, and Ries, Kristen (1996). "An Interdisciplinary, Interagency, Primary Care Approach to Case Management of the Dually Diagnosed Patient with HIV Disease." *Journal of the Association of Nurses in AIDS Care, 7*(5), pp. 72-82.

Chapter 2

Prochaska, James, Redding, Colleen, Harlow, L. L., Rossi, Joseph, and Velicer, Wayne (1994). "The Transtheoretical Model of Change and HIV Prevention: A Review." *Health Education Quarterly, 21*(4), pp. 471-486.

Chapter 4

Baum, Joanne (1985). *One Step Over the Line,* San Francisco: Harper & Row.
Hamilton, De Vance, Decker, Norman, and Rumbart, Ruben (1986). "The Manipulative Patient." *American Journal of Psychotherapy, 40*(2), pp. 189-200.
Hepworth, Dean (1993). "Managing Manipulative Behavior in the Helping Relationship." *Social Work, 38*(6), pp. 674-682.
Kirkham, Ann (1980. "Personality Disorders and Sexual Deviations." In Lancaster, Jeanette, *Adult Psychiatric Nursing,* New York: Medical Examination Publishing Co., Inc., pp. 273-327.

Chapter 6

King, Michael (1993). *AIDS, HIV, and Mental Health,* Cambridge, England: Cambridge University Press.

Chapter 7

Ashley, Rebecca, Carlson, Robert, Falck, Russell, and Seigal, Harvey (1995). "Injection Drug Users, Crack Cocaine Users, and Human Services Utilization." *Social Work, 40*(1), pp. 75-82.
Brennen, David and Dennis, Jeanne (1996). "Psychosocial Issues in HIV/AIDS Care." *Resource Manual for Providing Hospice Care to People Living with AIDS.* National Hospice Association, pp. 9-15.
Carr, Daniel and Addison, Robert (1994). "Pain in HIV/AIDS." Presented at a workshop convened by France-USA Pain Association, University of Strasbourg.
Jaffe, Jerome (1990). "Drug Addiction and Drug Abuse." In Gilman, A., Rall, T., Nies, A., and Taylor, P. (eds.), *Goodman and Gilman's the Pharmacological Basis of Therapeutics,* Eighth edition, New York: Pergamon Press.
King, Michael (1993). *AIDS, HIV, and Mental Health,* Cambridge, England: Cambridge University Press.

Chapter 8

Cull, Vera (1996). "Exposure to Violence and Self-Care Practices of Adolescents." *Family and Community Health, 19*(1), pp. 31-41.
Fontanarosa, Philip (1995). "The Unrelenting Epidemic of Violence in America. *Journal of American Medical Association, 273*(22), pp. 1792-1793.

Miller, David (1990). "Diagnosis and Treatment of Acute Psychological Problems related to HIV Infection and Disease." In Ostrow, David (ed.), *Behavioral Aspects of AIDS,* New York: Plenum, pp. 187-206.

Phillips, Kenneth (1996). "Extrapunitive and Intrapunitive Anger of HIV Caregivers: Nursing Implications." *Journal of the Association of Nurses in AIDS Care, 7*(2), pp. 17-26.

Seals, Brenda (1996). "The Overlapping Epidemics of Violence and HIV." *Journal of the Association of Nurses in AIDS Care, 7*(5), pp. 91-93.

Singer, Merrill (1994). "AIDS and the Health Crisis of the U.S. Urban Poor: The Perspective of Critical Medical Anthropology." *Social Science and Medicine, 39*(7), pp 931-948.

Wartenberg, Alan and Samet, Jeffrey, H. (1992). "The Drug-Using Patient." In Libman, Howard and Witzberg, Robert (eds.), *HIV Infection: A Clinical Manual,* Second edition. Boston: Little, Brown & Co., Inc., pp. 455-466.

Chapter 9

Marlin, Emily (1989). *Relationships in Recovery: Healing Strategies for Couples and Families,* New York: Harper & Row.

VandeCreek, Leon and Knapp, Samuel (1989). *Tarasoff and Beyond: Legal and Clinical Considerations in the Treatment of Life-Endangering Patients,* New York: Professional Resource Press.

Chapter 10

Mellors, John, Rinaldo, Charles, Gupta, Phalguni, White, R., Todd, John, and Kingsley, Lawrence (1996). "Prognosis in HIV-1 Infection Predicted by the Quantity of Virus in Plasma." *Science, 272*(11), pp. 57-70.

Statlanders Managed Pharmacy Services (1997). "Making Strides in the Fight Against AIDS." *Compliance Monitor,* Issue 2, p. 1.

Chapter 13

Byock, Ira (1994). "The Hospice Response to Euthanasia/Physician Assisted Suicide." *The Hospice Journal, 9*(4), p. 8.

Chapter 14

Woods, Joycelyn (1995). "How Methadone Works." *Basic Pharmacology.* Presented by the National Alliance of Methadone Advocates Educational Series No. 5, May. Available in AOL Netfind, www.methadone.org/hon.html.

Chapter 16

Nykanen, David, Kissoon, Niranjan, Rieder, Michael, and Armstrong, Ross (1991). "Comparison of a Topical Mixture of Lidocaine and Prilocaine

(ELMA, product of Astra Pharmaceuticals, Inc.) versus 1 Percent Lidocaine Infiltration on Wound Healing." *Pediatric Emergency Care, 7*(1), pp. 15-17.

Chapter 18

Katz, William (1993). *Minorities Today: A History of Multicultural America,* Austin, Texas: Raintree Steck-Vaughn Publishers.

Thernstrom, Stephan, Orlov, Ann, and Handlin, Oscar (eds.) (1980). *Harvard Encyclopedia of American Ethnic Groups*, Cambridge, MA: Harvard University Press, pp. 452-453; 458-460; 863-867.

Glossary

Acquired: Relating to a condition that is not inherited.

Acyclovir (Zovirax): An antiviral agent used to treat genital herpes.

AIDS: (Acquired Immunodeficiency Syndrome). A condition characterized by an impairment of the immune system that leaves affected individuals susceptible to certain cancers and opportunistic infections. Currently a diagnosis is made based on the presence of one or more diseases or conditions as defined by the Centers for Disease Control (CDC). The CDC has proposed expanding the definition of AIDS to include all HIV-infected individuals with T4 cell counts below 200 per measured unit of blood regardless of the presence of other diseases. (*See* CD4+)

Amphotericin B: An antifungal drug given to patients with cryptoccocal infection, histoplasmosis, or severe candidiasis. Side effects of the drug include fever, chills, kidney toxicity, anorexia, and vomiting.

Anemia: A condition in which there is a lower than normal number of red blood cells. Typical symptoms include headaches, drowsiness, and general malaise. Patients with severe anemia may require blood transfusions.

Anorectal condylomata: Uncomfortable lesions occurring on and within the anus and the rectum that are caused by a virus.

Anorexia: Loss of appetite that may result in significant weight loss.

Antibody: A protein substance developed by the body, usually in response to stimulation by an antigen. Antibodies destroy or neutralize bacteria, viruses, or other harmful toxins.

Antiretroviral therapy: Treatment aimed at destroying a virus or suppressing its disease-causing action.

Ascites: A complication of end-stage liver disease; an accumulation of fluid throughout the abdominal and pelvic areas.

AZT (zidovudine or Retrovir): An antiretroviral drug approved by the Food and Drug Administration (FDA) in 1987 that has been proven effective in reducing the rate of opportunistic infections and increasing life expectancy among individuals with HIV infection.

Bacteria: A single-cell organism that can cause certain diseases.

Bactrim (TMP/SMX): An antibiotic given for prophylaxis and treatment of *Pneumocystis carinii* pneumonia (PCP).

Cachexia: A profound state of ill health and malnutrition.

Candidiasis: A fungal infection that involves the skin (dermatocandidiasis), mouth (oral thrush), esophagus (candida esophagitis), respiratory tract (bronchocandidiasis), or vagina (vaginitis). Candidiasis of the esophagus and respiratory tract is an indicator disease for AIDS.

Case manager: person trained to act as an advocate and a connection to the legal and health care systems.

CD4+: The primary host cell infected by HIV; also known as T helper or T4 lymphocytes.

Contagious: Any infectious disease that can be transmitted casually from one person to another.

Cryptococcal meningitis: A fungal infection that causes inflammation of the spinal cord or brain. Typical symptoms include headaches, blurred vision, nausea, and confusion. Cryptococcal meningitis is one of the most frequent opportunistic infections in persons with AIDS.

Cytomegalovirus (CMV): A virus related to the herpes family. CMV infections may involve the eyes, central nervous system, lungs, and gastrointestinal tract. CMV can cause blindness in people with AIDS suffering from CMV-induced retinitis. The disease cannot be cured. Patients are treated with intravenous DHPG (ganciclovir). If treatment is withdrawn, symptoms will recur.

Dapsone: An antibiotic given in combination with AZT or pentamidine for acute treatment and prevention of PCP (*pneumocystis carinii* pneumonia). Side effects of the drug include anorexia, nausea, and vomiting.

ddC (Zalcitabine): An antiviral drug that can cause significant rises in CD4+ cell counts. However, approximately half of all patients receiving the drug have experienced reversible painful neuropathy.

ddI (Didanosine): An antiviral drug, tolerated by most patients and much less toxic than AZT.

Dementia: Chronic deterioration of an individual's mental capacity, including memory, perception, judgment, and language.

Diazepam (Valium): A medication prescribed to treat anxiety.

Edema: Swelling due to fluid retention.

Elavil (amitriptyline): An antidepressant often prescribed in AIDS to relieve painful peripheral neuropathy.

Electrolyte: A compound that, in solution, conducts electricity.

Epidemic: Affecting many individuals within a population, community, or region at the same time; an outbreak with sudden, rapid spread.

Erythromycin: An antibiotic prescribed to treat bacterial infections.

Esophagus: The tube connecting the oral cavity and the stomach.

Fluconazole (Diflucan): An antifungal drug given for prevention of fungal infections in advanced HIV infection as well as to treat active fungal infections such as candidiasis and cryptococcal meningitis.

Fungus: A potentially infectious organism that flourishes in dark, damp enviornments.

Haldol (haloperidol): An antipsychotic medication given to treat agitation.

Health care worker/provider: A person trained in any health-related field (for example: a case manager, certified nursing assistant, registered nurse, nurse practitioner, social worker, medical social worker, physician assistant, or physician).

Herpes Simplex Virus 1 (HSV-1): A virus that causes cold sores or fever blisters on the mouth, throat, or eyes and can be transmitted to the genital area. The latent virus can be reactivated by stress, other infections, or a compromised immune status.

Herpes Simplex Virus 2 (HSV-2): A virus that causes painful sores of the anus or genitals. It may lie dormant in nerve tissue and can be reactivated to produce the sores.

Herpes Varicella-Zoster Virus (HVZ): The reactivation of the varicella virus in adults, which is the same virus that causes chicken pox in children. Herpes zoster, also known as shingles, is characterized by very painful blisters on the skin following nerve pathways.

HIV seropositive: Showing antibodies as the result of infection with HIV.

Immune deficiency: A breakdown in an individual's immune system, making the individual susceptible to diseases that he or she would not ordinarily develop.

Intravenous drug user (IDU): Anyone who injects a drug directly into a vein.

Intravenous drugs: Drugs injected by needle directly into a vein.

Kaposi's sarcoma: A rare malignant skin tumor that occurs in some people with AIDS. Kaposi's sarcoma usually appears as purplish lesions on the skin but may also occur in the gastrointestinal tract, lymphatic system, lungs, or liver.

Medicaid: A state and federally funded, state-administered health insurance program for low-income persons.

Medicare: The federal health insurance program for the elderly, the permanently disabled, and individuals with end-stage kidney disease.

M S Contin: A slow-release narcotic (morphine) prescribed to treat a severe level of pain.

Mycobacterium Avium Intracellulare (MAI): A bacterial infection that can involve the gastrointestinal tract, lungs, bone marrow, or liver. MAI infections are common opportunistic infections of terminally ill AIDS patients. Symptoms may include fatigue, fever, night sweats, weight loss, and diarrhea.

Mycobutin (rifabutin): An antimicrobial prescribed to limit mycobacteria dissemination in patients with advanced HIV infection.

Neutropenia: An abnormally low neutrophil (white blood cell) count, which can leave a patient susceptible to bacterial and fungal infections.

Nonsteroidal anti-inflammatory drug (NSAID): A drug that decreases discomfort by reducing inflammation, which does not contain steroids. Available in low dose over the counter or in greater strengths by prescription.

Nystatin (Mycostatin): An antifungal liquid suspension usually swished around the oral cavity before being swallowed.

Opportunistic infection: An infection with any organisms that occurs when the host's immune system is compromised.

Pathogen: Any microorganism or virus that can cause disease.

Percocet (oxycodone): A combination narcotic and acetaminophen prescribed to treat a moderate level of pain unresponsive to milder medications.

Person/people living with AIDS (PLWA): Anyone diagnosed with the disease AIDS.

Peripheral neuropathy: Damage to the nerves in the feet, hands, or legs. Symptoms may include pain, numbness, and a tingling sensation.

***Pneumocystis carinii* pneumonia (PCP):** A severe, life-threatening lung infection found in 80 percent of all people with AIDS at some time during the course of their illness.

Primary caregiver: A person identified as willing and able to take on the responsibility for the needs of someone who is ill.

Prophylaxis: Treatment aimed at preserving health and preventing the spread of the disease.

Protease inhibitor: A class of drugs that interferes with the availability of the precursor for HIV replication and development.

Psychosocial: The relationship between the mind and the physical environment.

Seroconversion: Process by which a person's antibody status changes from negative to positive.

Social Security Insurance: Federal entitlement to a monthly payment for qualifying individuals.

STD: Sexually transmitted disease.

Syndrome: A group of symptoms that characterize a disease or condition.

Thrush: *See* Candidiasis.

Toxoplasmosis: A common opportunistic infection in persons with HIV infection.

Vicodin (hydrocodone): A combination drug of a mild narcotic and acetaminophen prescribed for treatment of a mild to moderate level of pain.

Virus: A potentially infectious organism; smaller in size than any other microorganism.

Bibliography

Anders, Gigi (1993). "Machismo: Dead or Alive?" *Hispanic, 6*(1), pp. 14-18.

Ashley, Rebecca, Carlson, Robert, Falck, Russell, and Seigal, Harvey (1995). "Injection Drug Users, Crack Cocaine Users, and Human Services Utilization." *Social Work 40*(1), pp. 75-82.

Baker, Nancy T. and Seager, Robert D. (1991). "Comparison of the Psychosocial Needs of Hospice Patients with AIDS and Those with Other Diagnoses." *The Hospice Journal, 7*(2), pp. 61-69.

Barlett, John A. (1996). *Care and Management of Patients with HIV Infection.* Durham, NC: GlaxoWellcome/Clean Data, Inc.

Baum, Joanne (1985). *One Step Over the Line.* San Francisco: Harper & Row.

Beresford, Larry (1993). *The Hospice Handbook.* New York: Little, Brown & Co.

Bly, Janet and Kissick, Priscilla (1994). "Hospice Care for Patients Living Alone: Results of a Demonstration Program." *The Hospice Journal, 9*(4), pp. 9-20.

Brennen, David and Dennis, Jeanne (1996). "Psychosocial Issues in HIV/AIDS Care." Resource Manual for Providing Hospice Care to People Living with AIDS. National Hospice Association, pp. 9-15.

Buckingham, Robert (1992). *Among Friends.* New York: Prometheus Books.

Byock, Ira (1994). "The Hospice Response to Euthanasia/Physician Assisted Suicide." *The Hospice Journal, 9*(4), p. 8.

Carr, Daniel and Addison, Robert (1994). "Pain in HIV/AIDS." Presented at a workshop convened by France-USA Pain Association, University of Strasbourg.

Carr, Gary (1996). "Ethnography of an HIV Hotel." *Journal of the Association of Nurses in AIDS Care, 7*(2), pp. 35-42.

Casey, Kathleen, Cohen, Felissa, and Hughes, Anne (1996). *ANAC's Core Curriculum for HIV/AIDS Nursing.* Philadelphia: Nursecom, Inc.

Cull, Vera (1996). "Exposure to Violence and Self-Care Practices of Adolescents." *Family and Community Health, 19*(1), pp. 31-41.

Day, Dawn (1997). "The Spread of Drug-Related AIDS Among African Americans and Latinos." *Health Emergency,* a pamphlet. Special Report by the Dogwood Center, Princeton, New Jersey.

Department of Health and Human Services (1997). "Needle Exchange Programs in America: Review of Published Studies and Ongoing Research." Report to the Committee on Appropriations for the Department of Labor, Health and Human Services, Education and Related Agencies, Washington, DC.

Duncan, David (1995). "A New Direction for Drug Education Harm Reduction." *The Catalyst* (New York State Federation of Professional Health Educators), *22*(2), pp. 8-9.

Duncan, David, Nickolson, Thomas, Clifford, Patrick, Hawkins, Wesley, and Petosa, Rick (1994). "Harm Reduction: An Emerging New Paradigm for Drug Education." *Journal of Drug Education, 24*(4), pp. 281-289.

Editorial (1998). "Needle Exchange Programmes in the USA: Time to Act Now." *The Lancet, 351,* p. 75.

Fitzgerald, Brianne, Aranda-Naranjo, Barbara, Ferri, Richard, and Deneberg, Risa (1996). "Applying the Transtheoretical and Harm Reduction Models." *Journal of the Association of Nurses in AIDS Care, 7*(1), pp. 33-40.

Flaskerud, Jacquelyn H. and Ungvarski, Peter (1995). *HIV/AIDS: A Guide to Nursing Care.* Philadelphia: W. B. Saunders Co.

Fleming, Michael and Barry, Kristen (1992). *Addictive Disorders*, St Louis, MO: Mosby Year Book Inc.

Fontanarosa, Philip (1995). "The Unrelenting Epidemic of Violence in America." *Journal of American Medical Association, 273*(22), pp. 1792-1793.

GlaxoWellcome (May/June, 1997), "HIV Care for Substance Users," *HIV Frontline.* A newsletter for professionals who counsel people with AIDS. Issue 28, p. 1.

Hamilton, De Vance, Decker, Norman, and Rumbart, Ruben (1986). "The Manipulative Patient." *American Journal of Psychotherapy, 40*(2), pp. 189-200.

Hepworth, Dean (1993). "Managing Manipulative Behavior in the Helping Relationship." *Social Work, 38*(6), pp. 674-682.

Jaffe, Jerome (1990). "Drug Addiction and Drug Abuse." In Gilman, Alfred, Rall, T., Nies, A., and Taylor, P. (eds.), *Goodman and Gilman's The Pharmacological Basis of Therapeutics,* Eighth edition, New York: Pergamon Press, pp. 522-573.

Kassinove, Howard and Sukhodolsky, Denis (1995). "Anger Disorders: Basic Science and Practice Issues." *Issues in Comprehensive Pediatric Nursing, 18*(3), pp. 173-205.

Katz, William (1993). *Minorities Today: A History of Multicultural America,* Austin, Texas: Raintree Steck-Vaughn Publishers.

King, Michael (1993). *AIDS, HIV, and Mental Health.* Cambridge, England: Cambridge University Press.

Kirkham, Ann (1980). "Personality Disorders and Sexual Deviations." In Lancaster, Jeanette, *Adult Psychiatric Nursing,* New York: Medical Examination Publishing Co., Inc., pp. 273-327.

Kovacs, Pamela and Rodgers, Antoinette (1995). "Meeting the Social Service Needs of Persons with AIDS: Hospices' Response." *The Hospice Journal, 10*(4), pp. 49-64.

Lurie, Peter and Drucker, Ernest (1997). "An Opportunity Lost: HIV Infections Associated with Lack of a National Needle Exchange Program in the USA." *The Lancet, 349,* pp. 604-608.

Lyons, Catherine (1996). "Harm Reduction in Practice: Applications in an HIV Clinic." Poster presentation at the ANAC Conference, Chicago, Illinois.

Marlin, Emily (1989). *Relationships in Recovery: Healing Strategies for Couples and Families.* New York: Harper & Row.

Mellors, John, Rinaldo, Charles, Gupta, Phalguni, White, R., Todd, John, and Kingsley, Lawrence (1996). "Prognosis in HIV-1 Infection Predicted by the Quantity of Virus in Plasma." *Science, 272*(11), pp. 57-70.

Mellors, John, Mulloz, Alvaro, Giorgi, Janis, Margolik, Joseph, Tassoni, Charles, Gupta, Phalguni, Kingsley, Lawrence, Todd, John, Saah, Alfred, Detels, Roger, Phair, John, and Rinaldo, Charles (1997). "Plasma Viral Load and CD4+ Lymphocytes as Prognostic Markers of HIV-1 Infection." *Annals of Internal Medicine, 126,* pp. 946-954.

Miller, David (1990). "Diagnosis and Treatment of Acute Psychological Problems related to HIV Infection and Disease." In Ostrow, David (ed.), *Behavioral Aspects of AIDS,* New York: Plenum, pp. 187-206.

Mount Sinai Hospital and Casey House Hospice (1995). *Module 4: Palliative Care: A Comprehensive Guide for the Care of Persons with HIV Disease.* Ferris, F. D., Flannery, J. S., McNeal, H. B., Morissette, M. R., Cameron, R., and Bally, G. A. (eds.), Toronto, Canada: Kirkpatrick & Associates Printing, Inc.

North American Syringe Exchange Network (1997). "Prevention as Politics." Presentation at the North American Syringe Exchange Convention, San Diego, CA.

Nykanen, David, Kissoon, Niranjan, Rieder, Michael, and Armstrong, Ross (1991). "Comparison of a Topical Mixture of Lidocaine and Prilocaine (Emla, product of Astra Pharmaceuticals, Inc.) versus 1 Percent Lidocaine Infiltration on Wound Healing." *Pediatric Emergency Care, 7*(1), pp. 15-17.

Peluso, Emanuel and Peluso, Lucy S. (1988). *Women & Drugs: Getting Hooked, Getting Clean.* Minneapolis: CompCare Publishers.

Phillips, Kenneth (1996). "Extrapunitive and Intrapunitive Anger of HIV Caregivers: Nursing Implications." *Journal of the Association of Nurses in AIDS Care, 7*(2), pp. 17-26.

Prochaska, James, Redding, Colleen, Harlow, L. L., Rossi, Joseph, and Velicer, Wayne. (1994). "The Transtheoretical Model of Change and HIV Prevention: A Review." *Health Education Quarterly, 21*(4), pp. 471-486.

Robb, Val (1994). "The Hotel Project: A Community Approach to Persons with AIDS." *Nursing Clinics of North America, 29*(3), pp. 521-531.

Rosenbaum, Marsha (1997). "Kids, Drugs, and Drug Education. A Harm Reduction Approach." Policy statement by the National Council on Crime and Delinquency. The Lindsmith Center, San Francisco, California.

Saag, Michael (1997). "Use of HIV Viral Load in Clinical Practice: Back to the Future." *Annals of Internal Medicine, 126* (12), pp. 983-985.

Seals, Brenda (1996). "The Overlapping Epidemics of Violence and HIV." *Journal of the Association of Nurses in AIDS Care, 7*(5), pp. 91-93.

Singer, Merrill (1994). "AIDS and the Health Crisis of the U.S. Urban Poor: The Perspective of Critical Medical Anthropology." *Social Science and Medicine, 39*(7), pp. 931-948.

Snyder, Carol, Kaempfer, Suzanne, and Ries, Kristen (1996). "An Interdisciplinary, Interagency, Primary Care Approach to Case Management of the Dually Diagnosed Patient with HIV Disease." *Journal of the Association of AIDS Care, 7*(5), pp. 72-82.

Springer-Bradley, Lucy (1996). "Patient Education for Behavior Change: Help from Transtheoretical and Harm Reduction Models." *Journal of the Association of Nurses in AIDS Care, 7*(1), pp. 23-32.

Statlanders Managed Pharmacy Services (1997). "Making Strides in the Fight Against AIDS." *Compliance Monitor,* Issue 2, p. 1.

Thernstrom, Stephan, Orlov, Ann, and Handlin, Oscar (eds.) (1980). *Harvard Encyclopedia of American Ethnic Groups*, Cambridge, MA: Harvard University Press, pp. 452-453; 458-460; 863-867.

VandeCreek, Leon and Knapp, Samuel. (1989). *Tarasoff and Beyond: Legal and Clinical Considerations in the Treatment of Life-Endangering Patients*. New York: Professional Resource Press.

Wartenberg, Alan and Samet, Jeffrey, H. (1992). *The Drug-Using Patient*. In Libman, Howard and Witzburg, Robert (eds.), *HIV Infection: A Clinical Manual*, Second edition, Boston: Little, Brown & Co., Inc., pp. 455-466.

Woods, Joycelyn (1997). "How Methadone Works." *Basic Pharmacology*. Presented by the National Alliance of Methadone Advocates Educational Series, No. 5, May. Available in AOL Netfind, www.methadone.org/how.html.

Zevin, Barry (1997). "HIV Care for Substance Users." *HIV Frontline, 28*, pp. 3-4.

Zierler, S., Witbeck, B., and Mayer, K. (1996). "Sexual Violence Against Women Living with or at Risk for HIV Infection." *American Journal of Preventive Medicine, 12*, pp. 204-210.

Index

Order Your Own Copy of
This Important Book for Your Personal Library!

HIV/AIDS AND THE DRUG CULTURE
Shattered Lives

_____ in hardbound at $39.95 (ISBN: 0-7890-0465-8)

_____ in softbound at $19.95 (ISBN: 0-7890-0554-9)

COST OF BOOKS _____

OUTSIDE USA/CANADA/
MEXICO: ADD 20% _____

POSTAGE & HANDLING _____
*(US: $3.00 for first book & $1.25
for each additional book)
Outside US: $4.75 for first book
& $1.75 for each additional book)*

SUBTOTAL _____

IN CANADA: ADD 7% GST _____

STATE TAX _____
*(NY, OH & MN residents, please
add appropriate local sales tax)*

FINAL TOTAL _____
*(If paying in Canadian funds,
convert using the current
exchange rate. UNESCO
coupons welcome.)*

☐ **BILL ME LATER:** ($5 service charge will be added)
(Bill-me option is good on US/Canada/Mexico orders only;
not good to jobbers, wholesalers, or subscription agencies.)

☐ Check here if billing address is different from
shipping address and attach purchase order and
billing address information.

Signature _____

☐ **PAYMENT ENCLOSED: $** _____

☐ **PLEASE CHARGE TO MY CREDIT CARD.**

☐ Visa   ☐ MasterCard   ☐ AmEx   ☐ Discover

Account # _____

Exp. Date _____

Signature _____

Prices in US dollars and subject to change without notice.

NAME _____

INSTITUTION _____

ADDRESS _____

CITY _____

STATE/ZIP _____

COUNTRY _____ COUNTY (NY residents only) _____

TEL _____ FAX _____

E-MAIL_____
May we use your e-mail address for confirmations and other types of information? ☐ Yes   ☐ No

Order From Your Local Bookstore or Directly From
The Haworth Press, Inc.
10 Alice Street, Binghamton, New York 13904-1580 • USA
TELEPHONE: 1-800-HAWORTH (1-800-429-6784) / Outside US/Canada: (607) 722-5857
FAX: 1-800-895-0582 / Outside US/Canada: (607) 772-6362
E-mail: getinfo@haworth.com
PLEASE PHOTOCOPY THIS FORM FOR YOUR PERSONAL USE.

BOF96

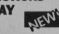

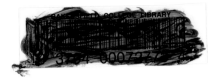
	DATE DUE		